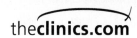

PHYSICAL MEDICINE AND REHABILITATION CLINICS OF NORTH AMERICA

Neuromuscular Complications of Systemic Conditions

GUEST EDITOR
Kathryn A. Stolp, MD

CONSULTING EDITOR
George H. Kraft, MD, MS

February 2008 • Volume 19 • Number 1

SAUNDERS

An Imprint of Elsevier, Inc.
PHILADELPHIA   LONDON   TORONTO   MONTREAL   SYDNEY   TOKYO

W.B. SAUNDERS COMPANY
A Division of Elsevier Inc.

1600 John F. Kennedy Blvd. • Suite 1800 • Philadelphia, Pennsylvania 19103

http://www.theclinics.com

PHYSICAL MEDICINE AND REHABILITATION
CLINICS OF NORTH AMERICA
February 2008
Editor: Debora Dellapena

Volume 19, Number 1
ISSN 1047-9651
ISBN 1-4160-5818-4
978-1-4160-5818-2

The ideas and opinions expressed in *Physical Medicine and Rehabilitation Clinics of North America* do not necessarily reflect those of the Publisher. The Publisher does not assume any responsibility for any injury and/or damage to persons or property arising out of or related to any use of the material contained in this periodical. The reader is advised to check the appropriate medical literature and the product information currently provided by the manufacturer of each drug to be administered to verify the dosage, the method and duration of administration, or contraindications. It is the responsibility of the treating physician or other health care professional, relying on independent experience and knowledge of the patient, to determine drug dosages and the best treatment for the patient. Mention of any product in this issue should not be construed as endorsement by the contributors, editors, or the Publisher of the product or manufacturers' claims.

Physical Medicine and Rehabilitation Clinics of North America (ISSN 1047-9651) is published quarterly by Elsevier Inc., 360 Park Avenue South, New York, NY 10010-1710. Months of publication are February, May, August, and November. Business and Editorial Offices: 1600 John F. Kennedy Blvd., Suite 1800, Philadelphia, PA 19103-2899. Customer Service Office: 6277 Sea Harbor Drive, Orlando, FL 32887-4800. Periodicals postage paid at New York, NY and additional mailing offices. Subscription price per year is $197.00 (US individuals), $308.00 (US institutions), $99.00 (US students), $240.00 (Canadian individuals), $394.00 (Canadian institutions), $135.00 (Canadian students), $277.00 (foreign individuals), $394.00 (foreign institutions), and $135.00 (foreign students). Foreign air speed delivery is included in all *Clinics* subscription prices. All prices are subject to change without notice. POSTMASTER: Send address changes to *Physical Medicine and Rehabilitation Clinics of North America*, Elsevier Periodicals Customer Service, 6277 Sea Harbor Drive, Orlando, FL 32887-4800. **Customer Service: 1-800-654-2452 (US). From outside of the US, call 1-407-345-4000.**

Physical Medicine and Rehabilitation Clinics of North America is indexed in *Excerpta Medica, Index Medicus, Cinahl,* and *Cumulative Index to Nursing and Allied Health Literature.*

Printed in the United States of America.

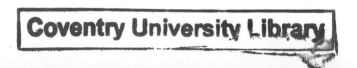

CONSULTING EDITOR

GEORGE H. KRAFT, MD, MS, Alvord Professor of Multiple Sclerosis Research; Professor, Rehabilitation Medicine; and Adjunct Professor, Neurology, University of Washington, School of Medicine, Seattle, Washington

GUEST EDITOR

KATHRYN A. STOLP, MD, Associate Professor, Chair, Mayo Clinic College of Medicine, Department of Physical Medicine and Rehabilitation, Mayo Clinic Rochester, Rochester, Minnesota

CONTRIBUTORS

SUNG C. AHN, DO, Assistant Professor, Loyola University, Maywood, Illinois

ANDREA J. BOON, MD, Assistant Professor, Department of Physical Medicine and Rehabilitation; Assistant Professor, Department of Neurology, Mayo College of Medicine, Mayo Clinic, Rochester, Minnesota

CHRISTIAN M. CUSTODIO, MD, Assistant Attending Physician, Department of Neurology, Rehabilitation Medicine Service, Memorial Sloan-Kettering Cancer Center; and Assistant Professor, Department of Rehabilitation Medicine, Joan and Sanford I. Weill Medical College of Cornell University, New York, New York

SHERILYN W. DRISCOLL, MD, Consultant, Director, Pediatric Physical Medicine and Rehabilitation, Mayo Clinic; Associate Professor, Mayo Clinic College of Medicine, Rochester, Minnesota

P. JAMES B. DYCK, MD, Head of the Peripheral Nerve Section and Professor of Neurology, Peripheral Neuropathy Research Laboratory, Mayo Clinic College of Medicine; Department of Neurology, Mayo Clinic, Rochester, Minnesota

BRENT P. GOODMAN, MD, Assistant Professor, Department of Neurology, Mayo College of Medicine; Co-Director, Electromyogram Laboratory, Mayo Clinic, Scottsdale, Arizona

CHARLENE HOFFMAN-SNYDER, NP-BC, CNP, Instructor of Neurology, Mayo Clinic College of Medicine, Department of Neurology, Mayo Clinic, Scottsdale, Arizona

E. WAYNE MASSEY, MD, Professor of Medicine, and Clinical Director of Muscular Dystrophy Clinics, Duke University, Department of Neurology, Duke University Medical Center, Durham, North Carolina

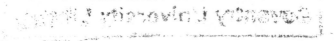

JESSICA ROBINSON-PAPP, MD, Assistant Professor, Departments of Neurology and Pathology, Mount Sinai Medical Center, New York, New York

DAVID M. SIMPSON, MD, Professor of Neurology, Director, Clinical Neurophysiology Laboratories and Neuro-AIDS Program, Department of Neurology, Mount Sinai Medical Center, New York, New York

JOLINE SKINNER, MD, Resident, Physical Medicine and Rehabilitation, Mayo Clinic, Rochester, Minnesota

BENN E. SMITH, MD, Associate Professor of Neurology, Mayo Clinic College of Medicine and Director of Electromyography Laboratory, Department of Neurology, Mayo Clinic, Scottsdale, Arizona

KATHRYN A. STOLP, MD, Associate Professor, Chair, Mayo Clinic College of Medicine, Department of Physical Medicine and Rehabilitation, Mayo Clinic Rochester, Rochester, Minnesota

PARIWAT THAISETTHAWATKUL, MD, Assistant Professor of Neurology, Department of Neurological Sciences, University of Nebraska Medical Center, Omaha, Nebraska

JENNIFER A. TRACY, MD, Peripheral Nerve Fellow, Peripheral Neuropathy Research Laboratory, Mayo Clinic College of Medicine; Department of Neurology, Mayo Clinic, Rochester, Minnesota

FAREN H. WILLIAMS, MD, MS, RD, Director of Physiatry, Clinical Professor, Department of Orthopedics and Physical Rehabilitation, University of Massachusetts Memorial, Worcester, Massachusetts

CONTENTS

> Diabetes mellitus is associated with many different neuropathic syndromes, ranging from a mild sensory disturbance as can be seen in a diabetic sensorimotor polyneuropathy, to the debilitating pain and weakness of a diabetic lumbosacral radiculoplexus neuropathy. The etiology of these syndromes has been studied extensively, and may vary among metabolic, compressive, and immunological bases for the different disorders, as well as mechanisms yet to be discovered. Many of these disorders of nerve appear to be separate conditions with different underlying mechanisms, and some are caused directly by diabetes mellitus, whereas others are associated with it but not caused by hyperglycemia. This article discusses a number of the more common disorders of nerve found with diabetes mellitus. It discusses the symmetrical neuropathies, particularly generalized diabetic polyneuropathy, and then the focal or asymmetrical types of diabetes-associated neuropathy.

> Death rates related to cancer have steadily decreased over the past few decades, and as a result, the number of survivors has exponentially increased. Increasingly, more and more secondary complications caused by cancer and its treatments are being recognized. Neuromuscular complications related to the

underlying cancer itself, or caused by associated treatments, such as chemotherapy and radiation therapy, are common but are likely underreported. While neurologic involvement can occur in both the central and peripheral nervous systems at any level, this article focuses on the effects of cancer on the peripheral nervous system.

Neuromuscular Complications of Statins

Sung C. Ahn

Statins, 3-hydroxy-3-methlglutaryl coenzyme A reductase inhibitors, are commonly prescribed for patients who have hyperlipidemia. Statins were first approved in 1987. Statin therapy is well documented to reduce serum low-density lipoprotein levels, incidence of cardiovascular events, and mortality. Although statin therapy is well tolerated, serious adverse affects have been reported, including neuromuscular and hepatic complications. Myopathy is particularly concerning because of the potential for rhabdomyolysis and death. Recently, peripheral neuropathy also has been identified as a possible complication. The incidence of neuromuscular complications is expected to increase with the increased number of people using statin therapy. Clinicians should be aware of the potential neuromuscular complications. This article reviews epidemiology, possible mechanisms, risk factors, and management of statin-associated neuromuscular complications.

Neuromuscular Disorders Associated with Paraproteinemia

Charlene Hoffman-Snyder and Benn E. Smith

Neuromuscular disorders associated with monoclonal gammopathies are usually uncovered in approximately 10% of patients presenting with peripheral neuropathy complaints. This discovery should prompt further evaluation for underlying plasma cell dyscrasias. The most frequent monoclonal disorders associated with neuropathy are smoldering myeloma, multiple myeloma, Waldenström macroglobulinemia, solitary plasmacytoma, systemic immunoglobulin light chain (AL) amyloidosis, POEMS (polyneuropathy, organomegaly, endocrinopathy, monoclonal gammopathy, and skin changes), and cryoglobulinemia. If these are excluded by careful evaluation the patient is classified as having monoclonal gammopathy of undetermined significance. Diagnostic criteria, risk stratification to determine prognosis, and current management for these disorders are reviewed in this article.

Neuromuscular Complications of Human Immunodeficiency Virus Infection

Jessica Robinson-Papp and David M. Simpson

Neurologic complications of HIV infection are common, and are a significant source of morbidity. The chronic nature of HIV today, the complexity of highly active antiretroviral therapy regimens, and the multiple and diffuse effects of HIV on the nervous system present an exciting diagnostic challenge, in which a systematic, comprehensive approach to diagnosis and treatment is necessary.

various ways during gestation. Quick recognition and treatment efforts should therefore be the clinician's goal. This article reviews peripheral neuropathy in pregnancy.

Musculoskeletal Complications of Neuromuscular Disease in Children

Sherilyn W. Driscoll and Joline Skinner

A wide variety of neuromuscular diseases affect children, including central nervous system disorders such as cerebral palsy and spinal cord injury; motor neuron disorders such as spinal muscular atrophy; peripheral nerve disorders such as Charcot-Marie-Tooth disease; neuromuscular junction disorders such as congenital myasthenia gravis; and muscle fiber disorders such as Duchenne's muscular dystrophy. Although the origins and clinical syndromes vary significantly, outcomes related to musculoskeletal complications are often shared. The most frequently encountered musculoskeletal complications of neuromuscular disorders in children are scoliosis, bony rotational deformities, and hip dysplasia. Management is often challenging to those who work with children who have neuromuscular disorders.

FORTHCOMING ISSUES

RECENT ISSUES

VISIT OUR WEB SITE

The Clinics are now available online!
Access your subscription at www.theclinics.com

ELSEVIER
SAUNDERS

Phys Med Rehabil Clin N Am
19 (2008) xi–xii

PHYSICAL MEDICINE
AND REHABILITATION
CLINICS OF
NORTH AMERICA

Foreword

Neuromuscular Complications of Systemic Conditions

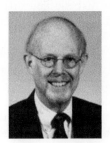

George H. Kraft, MD
Consulting Editor

During my training I was fascinated with the way in which many diseases affect the nervous system. As an electromyographer-in-training, I studied the effect of diabetes on the peripheral nervous system (frequently a neuropathy was present at the time of initial diagnosis) [1] and the pattern of demyelination with antigenic challenge (injected homogenized peripheral nerve could produce a monophasic model of Guillain-Barre syndrome in experimental animals) [2,3]. Later I was intrigued with the paraneoplastic effect: destruction of the nervous system produced by an immune attack from a distant tumor [4,5].

At that time—and I believe continuing through to the present day—the mecca for research on neuromuscular complications of systemic conditions was and continues to be the Mayo Clinic in Rochester, Minnesota. Over the years, physicians on the staff at Mayo, as well as their legion of residents and fellows, have identified, quantified, and studied these conditions. One of the best-known examples of this site expertise is the eponymous Lambert-Eaton syndrome, popularized in electrodiagnostic medicine circles by the late Ed Lambert.

It is in this tradition that I am grateful to Dr. Kathryn Stolp for having accepted an invitation to be the guest editor of an issue of the *Physical Medicine and Rehabilitation Clinics* on the neuromuscular complications of systemic conditions.

doi:10.1016/j.pmr.2007.10.011
pmr.theclinics.com

As practicing physicians—and often electromyographers—we are frequently faced with patients whose symptoms involve the peripheral and central nervous systems. The etiology may not be immediately obvious, but we are curious. The patient is referred to us for first confirming that there is, indeed, an abnormality of the nervous system; second, an assessment of where and how bad; and third, likely causes.

Dr. Stolp has drawn on the expertise of her colleagues at the Mayo Clinic and other affiliations to help us through this diagnostic and therapeutic maze. What is the latest on diabetic neuropathies? What does cancer do to the nervous system? And what about the effect of the various drugs in use today? Then there is HIV; what does it do the human nervous system? How about critical illness? What is the latest about the paraproteinemias? And how about nutritional deficiencies—dietary or acquired by bariatric surgery? Finally, how does pregnancy affect the neuromuscular system and what about pediatric neuromuscular diseases?

This is an exciting issue of the *Clinics*. It answers many of the questions that the reader may face in a practice of electrodiagnostic/rehabilitation medicine, and informs the reader about the latest in understanding of the causative links. Only the Mayo group could so competently answer these important and practical questions. My thanks to Kate Stolp and her distinguished colleagues. This issue of the *Clinics* will make for definitive answers to complex and baffling—but important and not infrequently encountered—questions for practicing physicians.

George H. Kraft, MD
Alvord Professor of MS Research
Professor Rehabilitation Medicine
Adjunct Professor, Neurology
University of Washington
1959 NE Pacific Street
Box 356490
Seattle, WA 98195-6490, USA

E-mail address: ghkraft@u.washington.edu

References

[1] Kraft GH, Guyton JD, Huffman JD. Follow-up study of motor nerve conduction velocities in diabetes mellitus. Arch Phys Med Rehabil 1970;51:207–9.
[2] Kraft GH. Experimental allergic neuritis: a model of idiopathic (Guillain-Barre) polyneuritis. Arch Phys Med Rehabil 1968;49:490–501.
[3] Kraft GH. Serial motor nerve latency and electromyography's determinations in experimental allergic neuritis. Electromyography 1971;11:61–74.
[4] Oei ME, Kraft GH, Sarnat HB. Intravascular lymphomatosis. Muscle Nerve 2002;25:742–6.
[5] Georgian-Smith D, Ellis GK, Kraft GH. Ampyiphysis paraneoplastic syndrome: a delayed diagnosis of breast carcinoma. Breast J 2003;9(4):316–8.

Phys Med Rehabil Clin N Am
19 (2008) xiii–xiv

PHYSICAL MEDICINE
AND REHABILITATION
CLINICS OF
NORTH AMERICA

Preface

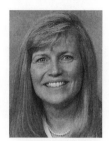

Kathryn A. Stolp, MD
Guest Editor

I thank Dr. George Kraft for inviting me to serve as guest editor for this issue of *Physical Medicine and Rehabilitation Clinics of North America*. The last two issues to discuss electrodiagnosis and neuromuscular diseases were published 10 and 5 years ago, respectively, and focused on the more technical aspects of patient evaluation. To complement these past issues, I have explored the challenges posed by various systemic conditions that, not uncommonly, result in disorders of nerve and muscle.

The articles in this issue review old conditions with new twists. Diabetes mellitus has well-known and well-documented neuromuscular complications, but there is a new understanding of pathoetiology and hence, new treatment recommendations. Though critical illness is well-known, the nerve or muscle problems that develop with it have new highlights. Pregnancy, a very well known and prevalent "condition" is associated with a number of neuropathies, the best known being carpal tunnel syndrome. Today, more people are surviving cancer, and given this fact, live with neuromuscular complications that were not fully recognized in the past. Patients who experience neuromuscular complications with human immune deficiency virus infections and paraproteinemias are also reviewed.

New neuromuscular disorders resulting from new medical and surgical treatments are also added to these most familiar conditions. In today's practice, health care providers will likely encounter problems resulting from treatment with cholesterol-lowering agents and surgery for obesity. Bariatric surgery results in neuromuscular complications from nutritional related and other events. In addition, a new understanding of nutritional deficiencies,

doi:10.1016/j.pmr.2007.10.007

their etiologies, and treatments are worth updating. Finally, how do we handle children who have neuromuscular disease, in this era of improved genetic analysis and management?

I thank everyone who contributed to this issue for not only their hard work and timely submissions, but also for sharing their knowledge and expertise. I hope you enjoy this issue.

Kathryn A. Stolp, MD
Department of Physical Medicine and Rehabilitation
Mayo Clinic
200 First Street SW
Rochester, MN 55905, USA

E-mail address: stolp.kathryn@mayo.edu

ELSEVIER
SAUNDERS

Phys Med Rehabil Clin N Am
19 (2008) 1–26

PHYSICAL MEDICINE
AND REHABILITATION
CLINICS OF
NORTH AMERICA

The Spectrum of Diabetic Neuropathies

Jennifer A. Tracy, MD[a,b], P. James B. Dyck, MD[a,b,*]

[a]*Peripheral Neuropathy Research Laboratory, Mayo Clinic College of Medicine,
200 First Street Southwest, Rochester, MN, USA*
[b]*Department of Neurology, Mayo Clinic, 200 First Street Southwest,
Rochester, MN 55905, USA*

The association between diabetes mellitus (DM) and neuropathy has been recognized for over 100 years, and soon it was realized that different subtypes existed, and so the first classification was proposed by Leyden [1] in 1893, with hyperesthetic (painful), paralytic (motor), and ataxic forms of diabetic neuropathy. There are many varieties of neuropathy classified under the term diabetic neuropathy, some clearly linked to hyperglycemia and subsequent metabolic and ischemic change, others with compressive etiologies, and still others associated with inflammatory/immune processes. Many types of nerves can be affected, including large-fiber sensory, small-fiber sensory, autonomic, and motor, and findings may or may not be symmetric. Distal nerves and nerve trunks, nerve roots, and cranial nerves can be damaged. The most common of these syndromes is the diabetic sensorimotor polyneuropathy, which can produce mild distal sensory abnormalities and distal weakness. Some of the rarer associated conditions, such as diabetic lumbosacral radiculoplexus neuropathy, are important to recognize, however, as they can produce severe pain and weakness with considerable morbidity. Prognoses for the diabetic neuropathy syndromes are also varied and dependent on the underlying pathology, with some of them being progressive disorders and others being monophasic illnesses. This article first discusses the more diffuse neuropathic processes, and then the focal and asymmetrical forms. Since Leyden's original classifications, many different classifications of diabetic neuropathy have been made. The two ways of classification preferred here are to divide diabetic

Supported in part by a grant obtained from the National Institute of Neurological Disease and Stroke (NINDS 36797).

* Corresponding author. Peripheral Neuropathy Research Laboratory, Mayo Clinic College of Medicine, 200 First Street Southwest, Rochester, MN.

E-mail address: dyck.pjames@mayo.edu (P.J.B. Dyck).

neuropathies by the clinical pattern into symmetrical or asymmetrical forms (Box 1) or to divide diabetic neuropathies based on the current understanding of pathophysiology (Table 1).

Diabetic sensorimotor polyneuropathy

DPN is felt to result from nerve and blood vessel changes caused by chronic hyperglycemic exposure, and this can occur in either type 1 or type 2 diabetics. This syndrome typically presents as a slowly progressive primarily sensory deficit in a length-dependent fashion, with symptoms starting in the feet and spreading upwards, evoking the classic stocking-glove distribution. In more severe cases, it will involve motor fibers also, and can produce footdrop and other distal lower extremity weakness. It can involve both large and small fibers, and can have associated autonomic

---

Box 1. Neuropathies associated with diabetes mellitus based on anatomical pattern

Symmetric
Diabetic polyneuropathy (DPN)
Diabetic autonomic neuropathy (DAN)
Neuropathy with impaired glucose tolerance
Painful sensory neuropathy with weight loss, (diabetic cachexia)
Insulin neuritis
Hypoglycemic neuropathy
Polyneuropathy after ketoacidosis
Chronic inflammatory demyelinating polyradiculoneuropathy
   in DM

Asymmetric
Diabetic cranial neuropathy
Diabetic mononeuropathy:
   Median neuropathy at the wrist
   Ulnar neuropathy at the elbow
   Peroneal neuropathy at the fibular head
Diabetic radiculoplexus neuropathies (DRPN)
Diabetic thoracic radiculoneuropathy (DTRN)
Diabetic lumbosacral radiculoplexus neuropathy (DLRPN)
Diabetic cervical radiculoplexus neuropathy (DCRPN)

Reprinted from Sinnreich M, Taylor BV, Dyck PJB. Diabetic neuropathies classification, clinical features, and pathophysiological basis. The Neurologist 2005;11(2):63–79; with permission.

Table 1
Pathophysiologic classification of diabetic neuropathies

Presumed underlying pathophysiology	Subtype of neuropathy
Metabolic-microvascular-hypoxic	Diabetic polyneuropathy
	Diabetic autonomic neuropathy
Inflammatory immune	Diabetic lumbosacral radiculoplexus neuropathy
	Diabetic thoracic radiculoneuropathy
	Diabetic cervical radiculoplexus neuropathy
	Cranial neuropathies
	Painful neuropathy with weight loss, (diabetic cachexia)
	Chronic inflammatory demyelinating polyradiculoneuropathy in diabetes mellitus
Compression and repetitive injury	Median neuropathy at the wrist
	Ulnar neuropathy at the elbow
	Peroneal neuropathy at the fibular head
Complications of diabetes	Neuropathy of ketoacidosis
	Neuropathy of chronic renal failure
	Neuropathy associated with large vessel ischemia
Treatment related	Insulin neuritis
	Hyperinsulin neuropathy

Reprinted from Sinnreich M, Taylor BV, Dyck PJB. Diabetic neuropathies classification, clinical features and pathophysiological basis. The Neurologist 2005;11(2):63–79; with permission.

symptoms and signs. Upper extremity symptoms/signs can appear as part of the proximal progression of deficits, but in most cases, these are caused by superimposed mononeuropathies (median neuropathy at the wrist and ulnar neuropathy at the elbow) rather than spread of the underlying polyneuropathy [2,3].

Dyck and colleagues evaluated 380 patients in a cohort of diabetic patients representative of the community (the Rochester Diabetic Neuropathy Study) and found that 66% of the patients with type 1 and 59% of the patients with type 2 DM had some type of neuropathy. In both the type 1 and type 2 patients, the most common neuropathy found was a DPN (the second most common neuropathy found in both of these groups was carpal tunnel syndrome). Despite the finding that DPN occurs commonly, most cases were asymptomatic and detected because of findings on clinical examination and electrophysiologic studies. Only 15% of the type 1 patients and 13% of the type 2 patients had a symptomatic polyneuropathy, and a very small percentage overall (6% of type 1 patients and 1% of type 2 patients) had severe symptomatic polyneuropathy with inability to walk on heels. These observations underscore the fact that most DPN is mild and that severe weakness only rarely occurs. In diabetic patients who have significant weakness, careful attention must be paid to other possible etiologies for their weakness, which can include other forms of diabetes-associated neuropathies, such as DLRPN (to be discussed later), and other types of neuromuscular disease that can occur independently of DM.

It has been shown that there are progressive subclinical nerve conduction abnormalities that precede the ultimate clinical diagnosis of DPN [4]. Gregersen [5] found a correlation between slowing of conduction velocities and duration of DM. A longitudinal study of risk factors for the severity of DPN found a correlation between severity and multiple other microvascular complications of diabetes such as retinopathy, proteinuria and microalbuminuria, and glycosylated hemoglobin. There was a strong correlation between the length of exposure of hyperglycemia and the degree of neuropathy (Fig. 1), and between the degree of neuropathy and degree of retinopathy (Fig. 2) [6,7].

The etiology of DPN seems to relate to microvascular damage. The cause of the microvascular damage may be multifactorial but probably relates to chronic hyperglycemia-mediated direct metabolic effect. Sural nerve biopsies of diabetic patients who have peripheral neuropathy reveal increased numbers of endothelial nuclei and excess thickness of endoneurial microvessels caused by reduplication of the endothelial basement membrane (Fig. 3), with a greater range in the thickness of vessel lumens [8]. There is also macrovascular disease that is probably the cause of coronary artery disease and stroke, which is found in nerves but is not the cause of DPN (Fig. 4).

Because of the significant morbidity that can occur with DPN and its association with hyperglycemia, there has been considerable interest in the

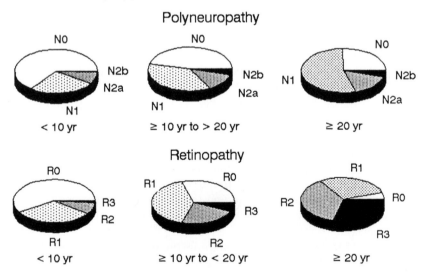

Fig. 1. The change in the stage distribution of neuropathy (*top*) and retinopathy (*bottom*) with increasing duration of diabetes mellitus. N0, no neuropathy; N1, subclinical neuropathy; N2a, symptomatic neuropathy, mild; N2b, symptomatic neuropathy, more severe; R0, no retinopathy; R1, early nonproliferative retinopathy; R2, late nonproliferative retinopathy; R3, proliferative retinopathy. (*Reprinted from* Dyck PJ, Kratz KM, Karnes JL, et al. The prevalence by staged severity of various types of diabetic neuropathy, retinopathy, and nephropathy in a population-based cohort: The Rochester Diabetic Neuropathy Study. Neurology 1993;43:817–24; with permission.)

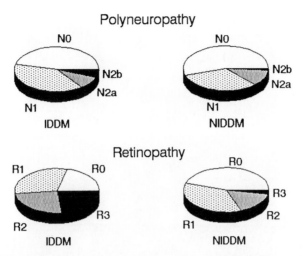

Fig. 2. A diagrammatic representation of Rochester, Minn., diabetic patients with insulin-dependent diabetes mellitus (IDDM, left) and noninsulin-dependent diabetes mellitus (NIDDM, right) who had different stages of severity of neuropathy (*top*) and retinopathy (*bottom*). For both complications, there is a more severe distribution of stages of the complication in IDDM than NIDDM. (*Reprinted from* Dyck PJ, Kratz KM, Karnes JL, et al. The prevalence by staged severity of various types of diabetic neuropathy, retinopathy, and nephropathy in a population-based cohort: The Rochester Diabetic Neuropathy Study. Neurology 1993;43:817–24; with permission.)

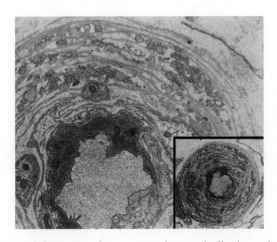

Fig. 3. This microvessel shows severe basement membrane reduplication and a very high number of cellular debris among the basement membrane leaflets. Basement membrane leaflets are often incomplete and fragmented. (× 14,000 before 25% reduction; inset, × 3600 before 25% reduction) (*From* Giannini C, Dyck PJ. Ultrastructural morphometric abnormalities of sural nerve endoneurial microvessels in diabetes mellitus. Ann Neurol 1994;36:408–15; with permission. Copyright © 1994, Wiley-Liss, Inc., A Wiley Company.)

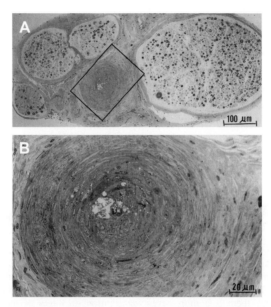

Fig. 4. Epineurial arterioles were more frequently abnormal in nerves of diabetics than in nerves of controls. (*A*) The arteriole enclosed by a rectangle. (*B*) Greater detail shows obliteration of the lumen by fat deposition, intimal proliferation, and thickening of the wall. (*From* Dyck PJ, Lais A, Karnes JL, et al. Fiber loss is primary and multifocal in sural nerves in diabetic polyneuropathy. Ann Neurol 1986;19:425–39; with permission. Copyright © 1986, Wiley-Liss, Inc., A Wiley Company.)

possibility of preventing, slowing, or reversing neuropathy by improved control of blood sugar. The Diabetes Control and Complications Trial Research Group studied 1441 insulin-dependent diabetic patients over a mean duration of 6.5 years and provided them with either conventional treatment, defined as one or two daily insulin injections, or intensive treatment, defined as at least three daily insulin injections or continuous insulin infusion with at least four glucose tests daily. They found that at 5 years, subjects receiving intensive therapy had a 64% less development of confirmed clinical neuropathy. Additionally, the prevalence of abnormal nerve conduction studies was lower by 44%, and abnormal autonomic function testing was lower by 53% in the intensively treated group [9]. This is an encouraging finding, and shows that good glycemic control can delay and probably prevent the development of DPN. There continue to be efforts to find neuroprotective agents that may be useful for treatment once DPN has occurred, however.

Because of growing evidence that oxidative damage may play a significant role in the development of polyneuropathy, antioxidant agents such as lipoic acid have been studied. In an experimental rat model of diabetic neuropathy (streptozotocin-induced), the administration of intraperitoneal lipoic acid improved nerve blood flow and markers of oxidative stress in a dose-dependent manner, and the conduction velocity of the digital nerve [10].

Alpha-lipoic acid was evaluated in human patients who had symptomatic DPN as part of the SYDNEY trial, in which patients were treated with either intravenous alpha-lipoic acid 5 days a week for a total of 14 treatments or placebo. The primary endpoint of change in total symptom score (TSS, which assesses positive neuropathic symptoms) was met by showing a significant improvement in positive symptoms in the treated group versus placebo. There was also a significant improvement in the neuropathy impairment score (NIS) [11]. The results of the ALADIN III study for alpha-lipoic acid were not as encouraging, however. This study randomized type 2 diabetic subjects who had DPN into three groups:

1. Alpha-lipoic acid intravenously daily for 3 weeks, then orally for 6 months
2. Alpha-lipoic acid intravenously daily for 3 weeks, then placebo orally for 6 months
3. Placebo intravenously daily for 3 weeks, then placebo orally for 6 months

In this study, which evaluated treatment effect for a longer period of time than the SYDNEY trial, there was no significant difference after 7 months between the groups in TSS and in change in NIS between the alpha-lipoic acid group and the placebo group [12].

There may be a role of increased activity of the polyol pathway and increased glycation end products in the pathogenesis of DPN [13]. Diabetic patients have been found to have higher levels of endoneurial glucose, fructose, and sorbitol than control patients [14]. There is greater overall microvessel area in nerve of streptozocin-induced diabetic rats, and microvessel basement membrane thickening has been prevented with the use of an aldose reductase inhibitor [15]. There are multiple trials studying the effects of various aldose reductase inhibitors, which block the polyol pathway, in an attempt to decrease or prevent the neuropathic complications of DM. Unfortunately, results have been mixed.

Judzewitsch and colleagues [16] used the aldose reductase inhibitor sorbinil in 39 diabetic patients, and found that there were very mild improvements in nerve conduction velocities after 9 weeks of treatment. The clinical significance of these slight changes is indeterminate. Another study of sorbinil in patients who had DPN used sorbinil or placebo for a 6-month period, and found no major differences in clinical benefit between the two groups, and no difference on sensory threshold studies. There was significant benefit in the sorbinil-treated group in only a very limited number of electrophysiologic and autonomic parameters, such as conduction velocity in the posterior tibial nerve [17]. Another aldose reductase inhibitor, tolrestat, was used to treat patients who had DPN over a 52-week period compared with placebo, and significant concordant improvement in paresthesias and motor nerve conduction velocities over placebo was found in the group receiving the highest tolrestat dose, 200 mg daily. Only 28% of the tolrestat-treated patients (at 200 mg/d), however, had concordant improvement at the 24-week evaluation maintained at the final 52-week evaluation [18]. Krentz and colleagues [19] treated patients with DPN with either ponalrestat, another aldose reductase inhibitor, or placebo for 52 weeks and found no significant differences between the groups in motor or sensory nerve conduction velocities, vibration thresholds, symptom scores, or autonomic function tests.

Recombinant human nerve growth factor (rhNGF), which promotes the survival of small fiber sensory and sympathetic neurons, also has been studied in patients who have DPN, with the hopes that it could improve impaired nerve function. Apfel and colleagues [20] performed a study in which 250 patients with symptomatic DPN were treated with 6 months of either rhNGF or placebo, and found a trend toward improvement in NIS(LL) in the treatment group. A trial evaluating the use of rhNGF in patients with HIV-associated sensory neuropathy found a benefit versus placebo in self-reported neuropathic pain intensity and pinprick sensitivity, suggesting that this may be a useful agent in different types of neuropathy [21]. These studies helped bolster enthusiasm for the potential benefit of this agent. A larger randomized, double-blind placebo-controlled trial of 1019 patients with either type 1 or type 2 diabetes and DPN administered either rhNGF or placebo over a 48-week period. No significant change between baseline and the 48-week examinations in the NIS(LL) was found [22].

These results are somewhat disheartening, and it remains unclear if any of these agents ultimately will be helpful in treating DPN. At present, control of blood sugars and prevention are the most important ways of dealing with DPN.

Diabetic autonomic neuropathy

Autonomic abnormalities can occur in DM with or without the presence of a large-fiber neuropathy. Many experts consider that DAN is really a part of the larger category of DPN. Low and colleagues [23] reviewed the autonomic symptoms and standardized autonomic testing of patients with DM (types 1 and 2) and of control patients, and found that 54% of patients with type 1 diabetes, and 73% of patients with type 2 diabetes had objective autonomic impairment, but this was generally in the mild range. Only 14% of the diabetic patients in that study had moderate-to-severe generalized autonomic failure. The numbers were even smaller for the Rochester Diabetic Neuropathy Study [7].

Autonomic failure can result in many troublesome symptoms, including orthostatic hypotension, nausea and constipation from abnormal gastrointestinal (GI) motility, incontinence, and erectile dysfunction. The complex management of each of these problems is beyond the scope of this discussion, and often requires the coordinated care of multiple medical specialties.

Autonomic instability in these patients may result in greater surgical risk and morbidity; Burgos and colleagues [24] prospectively studied 17 diabetic and 21 nondiabetic patients who had previously been given autonomic screening during elective ophthalmologic surgery and found that 35% of diabetics required intraoperative vasopressors compared with only 5% of the control group. Furthermore, the diabetics who required pressors had significantly greater autonomic impairment than those who did not. Investigators also have had concerns that DAN may be associated with sudden cardiac death, possibly related to abnormal lengthening of QT intervals [25]. A recent review of cases of sudden cardiac death in diabetic patients, however, has revealed a greater correlation between sudden cardiac death and atherosclerotic heart disease and nephropathy than with DAN. The authors conclude that although there is an association between autonomic neuropathy and sudden cardiac death in diabetic patients, it is probably not the causative factor, and atherosclerotic heart disease is more important [26].

Polyneuropathy associated with glucose intolerance

There is increasing interest in an association between impaired fasting glucose or impaired glucose tolerance (IGT), which does not meet the criteria for DM and the development of a chronic axonal polyneuropathy. Current American Diabetes Association (ADA) guidelines, recently revised in 2003, require a fasting plasma glucose from 100 mg/dL to 125 mg/dL, for a diagnosis of impaired fasting glucose, and a 2-hour glucose level from 140 mg/dL to 199 mg/dL (after a 75 g oral glucose load) for the diagnosis of IGT [27]. It is estimated that approximately 33% of adults in the United States over 60 years old have either DM or impaired fasting glucose (diagnosed or undiagnosed) [28]. This value was based on the earlier ADA criteria of impaired fasting glucose as a level between 110 mg/dL and 126 mg/dL, so the expectation is a higher overall incidence and prevalence with the new criteria. This percentage also does not take into account the greater number of patients with impaired glucose metabolism that may be detected through 2-hour oral glucose tolerance tests (OGTT), which would be expected to increase the purported population at risk. Studies have shown higher yields for abnormal glucose metabolism in glucose tolerance tests than in fasting plasma glucose measurements [29,30].

Singleton and colleagues [31] prospectively evaluated a cohort of 107 patients who had idiopathic symmetric distal peripheral neuropathy and found that 34% had IGT on an OGTT, which they noted was three times the prevalence of an age-matched historical cohort. Furthermore, only 72 of their subjects had an OGTT done, with a yield of 50% of the subjects receiving this test with an ultimate diagnosis of impaired glucose tolerance. The neuropathy pattern was predominantly sensory, as 81% of the patients with IGT had only sensory complaints, with 92% reporting neuropathic pain as a dominant symptom. Electrophysiologic findings revealed over half (61%) of the IGT patients had decreased sural sensory amplitudes, whereas only 21% had a decreased peroneal motor amplitude. Sumner and col-leagues [32] reported on 73 patients who had a peripheral neuropathy of un-known cause, and found that 56% of them had abnormal findings on an OGTT (26 of them with IGT and 15 with DM). The authors found that the patients with IGT had less severe neuropathy and more predominant small fiber involvement than the diabetic patients. Hoffman-Snyder and col-leagues [33] retrospectively assessed 100 consecutive patients with an idio-pathic chronic axonal neuropathy, who had fasting plasma glucose and a 2-hour OGTT. By the new ADA 2003 criteria, 39% of these patients had an abnormal fasting blood sugar, 36 of whom were in the range of im-paired fasting glucose, and three of whom were in the diabetic range. Using the OGTT, even a higher percentage (62%) of the patients had an abnormal glucose metabolism, 38 with IGT and 24 with DM. These rates were higher than previously published age-matched controls (33%) [28]. The authors commented that abnormal glucose metabolism was found at similar rates in sensorimotor, sensory, and small fiber neuropathies.

There is also some pathologic evidence of increased endoneurial capillary density in sural nerves of patients who have IGT progressing to DM com-pared with patients who have stable IGT, indicating that microvascular ab-normalities are occurring in a prediabetic state [34]. Skin biopsies of patients with neuropathy and IGT have demonstrated abnormal intraepidermal nerve fiber density [35,36]. Smith and colleagues [36] showed that patients who had IGT and neuropathy had significantly improved proximal intrae-pidermal nerve fiber density and improved response on OGTTs after 1 year of a diet and exercise counseling program compared with their base-line OGTTs. The authors noted, however, that patients who had absent dermal plexus on the initial biopsy were unlikely to have significant reinner-avation on repeat biopsy.

Not all evidence, however, has been supportive of the association between IGT and neuropathy. Eriksson and colleagues performed nerve conduction studies, heat, cold and vibration threshold testing, and auto-nomic function testing on patients who had IGT, diabetic patients, and nondiabetic controls. They found that aside from significantly more abnor-malities in heart rate with inspiration and expiration (suggestive of vagal nerve involvement), there were no other parameters that were significantly different between their patients with IGT and controls [37]. Hughes and col-leagues [38] studied 50 patients who had chronic idiopathic axonal polyneur-opathy and 50 control patients, with OGTT and fasting plasma glucose analysis, and did not find an association with IGT and neuropathy after ad-justing for age and sex. The lack of a significant association is particularly compelling, given that there was an active control group in the study, as op-posed to most of the other studies cited, which used historical control data as a comparative measure of prevalence of IGT in the general population.

At this point in time, the relationship between IGT and peripheral neuropathy needs further clarification. Although a very interesting and potentially important hypothesis, the association has not been proven definitely. A large epidemiology study has been begun looking at IGT and neuropathy in Olmsted County, Minn.

Acute painful diabetic neuropathy with weight loss

Cachexia and weight loss may be seen in association with DM [39]. This acute painful neuropathy with weight loss is considered by some authors to be a clinical entity separate from DPN [40,41]. This syndrome also is known as diabetic cachexia and is not related to the severity or duration of DM and has a monophasic course, usually over months. The illness begins with sudden, profound weight loss followed by severe pain, often burning, and excessive sensitivity to touch (allodynia) of the lower legs and feet. Autonomic features other than impotence are usually absent. Some experts have argued that this entity is part of the spectrum of DPN with the same underlying mechanism and pain fibers being predominantly involved. This monophasic course, the lack of correlation between DM duration, and the neuropathy with associated weight loss, make it unlikely to be part of DPN. In contrast, the occurrence of neuropathy in early DM, the associated weight loss, and the monophasic course are features that typically are found in DLRPN, which is described later . DLRPN has been shown to be caused by microvasculitis and ischemic injury. The pathological basis of acute painful diabetic neuropathy with weight loss has not been determined, but an immune mechanism seems likely.

Insulin neuritis

A rare form of peripheral neuropathy has been described in patients shortly after instituting insulin for DM, referred to as insulin neuritis. It first was described in 1933, but there have been multiple case reports of this phenomenon in the literature [42,43]. A typical example was that of a patient who had begun a continuous subcutaneous insulin infusion, and acutely developed a painful neuropathy. Sural nerve biopsy revealed changes of chronic neuropathy, and the authors raised the possibility that the symptoms were caused by abnormal ectopic sensory responses caused by axon regeneration [43]. Kihara and colleagues [44] evaluated the effect of insulin on nerve oxygenation in normal nerves and nerves of rats with streptozotocin-induced diabetes. They found that infusion of insulin caused a reduction in endoneurial oxygen tension in the normal nerves studied, and that streptozotocin-induced diabetic nerves were resistant to these changes. When the hyperglycemia in the diabetic nerves was controlled, however, they became more sensitive to this effect of insulin. As a result, nerve blood flow was decreased, and blood through arteriovenous shunts was increased. Tesfaye and colleagues [45] reviewed sural nerve epineurial vessel photography and fluorescein angiography of five patients who had insulin neuritis, and found severely abnormal epineurial vessels, with arteriovenous shunting and tortuosity, and in three patients proliferating leaky vessels were found. They suggested that perhaps these changes lead to an ischemic endoneurium. Recognition that immune factors are involved in other forms of diabetic neuropathy raises the possibility in insulin neuritis also.

Hypoglycemic neuropathy (hyperinsulinemic neuropathy)

There are several reports in the literature of polyneuropathy occurring in association with a chronic hyperinsulinemic state, and repeated episodes of hypoglycemia. This can be found in the context of an insulinoma, or insulin-secreting tumor of the pancreas.

Jaspan and colleagues [46] reviewed 29 of these cases in the literature, including a case of their own, and found a mean age of 38 years with a slight male predominance. The typical presentation was initially that of prominent distal uncomfortable paresthesias without significant objective sensory findings, followed by a motor-predominant distal symmetric peripheral neuropathy with atrophy. The upper extremities are generally more involved than the lower extremities, but foot drop is also common. Just less than half of the patients for whom detailed central nervous system (CNS) data were available showed some signs of CNS dysfunction, usually mental status or personality changes, although a small minority had cerebellar findings also. In their own case that they reported, both a sural nerve biopsy and a gastrocnemius biopsy were performed. A reduction in large myelinated fibers was observed on nerve biopsy, and muscle showed neurogenic atrophy, and a few necrotic fibers and some perivascular lymphocytes and histiocytes. Overall, in these patients, there was some improvement of weakness after removal of the insulinoma, and significant improvement of the sensory symptoms. They commented that peripheral nerve disease is rare compared with CNS disease in the hypoglycemic state, and that this may be related to the decreased dependence of the peripheral nervous system on glucose metabolism.

Westfall and colleagues [47] studied the effects of insulin in alloxan-induced diabetic rats, giving either daily insulin injections or insulin through a subcutaneous minipump. Controls were untreated diabetic rats and non-diabetic rats. Through teased fiber analysis of tibial nerves, they found evidence of Wallerian-type axonal degeneration only in the treated diabetic rats. Findings were worse in the daily insulin injection group, suggestive of primary damage to the nerves either through hyperinsulinemia or hypoglycemia. Sima and colleagues [48] studied hyperglycemic (diabetic biobred) rats, and gave them either small doses of insulin, high insulin doses to the point of hypoglycemia, or left them in a hyperglycemic state without insulin. In the hypoglycemic rats, loss of anterior horn cells, loss of large myelinated fibers, and decreased nerve conduction velocities were found, while the other groups had mainly sensory fiber abnormalities.

Although there is clearly evidence that hypoglycemia can damage peripheral nerve, the mechanism by which this happens is unclear. Also not clear is whether peripheral nerve damage occurs in diabetic patients who have intermittent periods of hypoglycemia, a topic that deserves further study.

Polyneuropathy after ketoacidosis

Diabetic ketoacidosis can present with profound CNS abnormalities, particularly a depressed level of consciousness [49]. A pathologic study of six patients who died with coma from diabetic ketoacidosis showed ischemic tissue damage both in the brain and other organs, felt to be related to abnormalities of intravascular coagulation [50]. There are limited reports of peripheral nervous system damage during periods of diabetic ketoacidosis, including the clinical picture of multiple mononeuropathies [51,52]. It is unclear if these changes result from peripheral nerve ischemia or other hemodynamic and metabolic abnormalities during the course of acute illness.

Chronic inflammatory demyelinating polyradiculoneuropathy in diabetes mellitus

Chronic inflammatory demyelinating polyradiculoneuropathy (CIDP), as its name suggests, is an immune-mediated disorder of the peripheral nervous system, with primary damage to the myelin sheath, although many patients will develop secondary axon loss over time. It is characterized by symmetric distal and proximal weakness, hyporeflexia, or areflexia, which progresses over at least a 2-month time period. Some people have a relapsing-remitting course, and others can have a progressive phenotype. It usually is accompanied by elevated cerebral spinal fluid protein and evidence of demyelination (slowed conduction velocities, temporal dispersion, conduction block, prolonged distal latencies, and prolonged F-wave latencies) on nerve conduction studies. Treatment is with immunomodulatory therapies, which can include steroids, intravenous immunoglobulin, plasma exchange, azathioprine, and a host of other immunosuppressive agents. There is suggestion in the literature that patients who have DM may be at increased risk to develop CIDP, although this has been studied incompletely [53]. Laughlin and colleagues [54] studied the incidence and prevalence of CIDP in the general population and among diabetic patients in Olmsted County, Minn., and did not find an increased frequency among diabetic patients. The authors noted that because the population they studied was small, minor association between DM and CIDP might be missed but that a large association was unlikely.

Gorson and colleagues [55] studied 14 patients who had DM and clinical and neurophysiologic findings of CIDP and compared them with 60 cases of idiopathic CIDP. Overall, the diabetic patients were older and had a greater occurrence of imbalance, but otherwise their clinical symptoms were not remarkably different from the patients who had idiopathic CIDP. Where they did differ is that on nerve conduction studies, the DM patients had significantly lower amplitude ulnar motor response; sural response was more likely to be absent, and there was a trend toward lower amplitude compound muscle action potential and sensory nerve action potential overall. In addition, the nerve biopsies of the diabetic patients were more likely to show predominately axonal loss than the CIDP patients. One explanation for these findings is that there is a superimposed DPN. The authors also noted that there was a lesser improvement in strength after immunomodulatory treatment in the DM group than the idiopathic CIDP. Stewart and colleagues [56] evaluated seven diabetic patients who had CIDP, and found that all had distal muscle chronic denervation changes and distal more than proximal weakness and wasting. Electrophysiologically, most had motor conduction block, slow conduction velocities, and prolonged distal latencies, and all had F-wave abnormalities. All received immunomodulatory treatment and had improvement of their symptoms; six of seven improved by at least two modified Rankin grades.

Although there is no question that diabetic patients can develop CIDP, the question remains whether DM is a risk factor for developing CIDP. One problem that exists in answering this question is that some authors have relied predominantly on nerve conduction studies in defining CIDP, and most other forms of diabetic neuropathy are known to have some demyelinating features on nerve conduction studies. Therefore, some cases of DPN (or other diabetic neuropathy) may be mislabeled as CIDP. Another potentially confusing group of conditions is comprised by the diabetic radiculoplexus neuropathies, which cause severe pain and weakness, and may be mislabeled as diabetic CIDP. These conditions also may respond to immune-modulating agents. Laughlin and colleagues [54] suggest, however, that if an association between diabetes and CIDP exists, it is small and probably not very clinically important. A definitive answer only can be obtained through large population-based studies. Regardless of an association, these studies provide a cautionary note about assuming that all neuropathies in a diabetic patient are caused solely by diabetes, as incomplete evaluation to identify other causes of neuropathy may deprive a patient of effective treatments, such as immunomodulatory therapy for CIDP.

Diabetic cranial neuropathy

Cranial neuropathies likely occur at a higher incidence in diabetic patients than in the general population, but this is insufficiently studied. Watanabe and colleagues [57] reviewed cranial nerve findings in 1961 diabetics and 3841 control subjects. He found a significantly higher incidence of cranial neuropathies (0.97%) in diabetic subjects than in the control subjects (0.13%), although the overall incidence was quite low in both groups.

The most common cranial neuropathies found were oculomotor nerve palsies and facial nerve palsies. In the Rochester Diabetic Neuropathy Study cohort, no patients presented with cranial neuropathies [7].

Diabetic oculomotor palsy typically presents acutely with severe eye pain and paresis of the oculomotor-innervated extraocular muscles: superior, inferior, medial rectus, and inferior oblique muscles. This is accompanied by ptosis from involvement of the levator palpebrae. In most cases, this is a pupil-sparing lesion, as the parasympathetic fibers travel in the peripheral layers of the nerve, and the putative mechanism in diabetic ophthalmoplegia is ischemic rather than compressive. Particularly, when there is pupillary involvement, alternative diagnoses such as enlarging aneurysm or other compressive lesions must be ruled out. The prognosis in diabetic oculomotor palsy is good, and full recovery generally occurs, although it may take months to regain normal function [58]. Other cranial nerves affecting extraocular muscles also can be involved in DM; in a study of 2229 patients who presented with an oculomotor palsy, 13.7% of them were found to be associated with DM. Of the diabetic group with cranial nerve involvement, 50% had cranial nerve VI involvement; 43.3% had cranial nerve III involvement, and 6.7% had cranial nerve IV involvement [59].

Facial nerve palsies are common in the general population, and it is unclear if their overall incidence is higher in the context of DM. As expected for a peripheral nerve lesion, this should result in weakness of the ipsilateral forehead and the rest of the ipsilateral face. There is no evidence that this should be treated in a different manner from idiopathic facial nerve palsy. Nerve conduction studies and electromyogram (EMG), including the blink reflex may be important for documenting nerve integrity and prognostication but generally are not needed for the diagnosis.

Diabetic mononeuropathies

Several mononeuropathies appear in greater frequency in diabetic patients than in the general population; these include median neuropathy at the wrist (carpal tunnel syndrome), ulnar neuropathy at the elbow, and peroneal neuropathy at the fibular head. As noted previously, most diabetic patients who have upper extremity neuropathic symptoms and signs will have a mononeuropathy or multiple mononeuropathies as the etiology rather than an extension of a generalized polyneuropathy [2,3].

Median neuropathy at the wrist, or carpal tunnel syndrome, can present with dysesthetic symptoms or numbness in the first three fingers of the hand and the lateral surface of the fourth finger, and/or weakness in median-innervated muscles of the hand. Sensory symptoms can extend into the wrist and forearm. There are many risk factors identified in the literature for development of carpal tunnel syndrome; these include rheumatoid arthritis, osteoarthritis of the wrist, previous wrist fracture, obesity, and diabetes

[60]. Of 414 patients with mild diabetic neuropathy enrolled for the EDIT trial, 23% met criteria for median neuropathy at the wrist (MNW). These patients overall had a longer duration of diabetes than patients without MNW. The authors also found that degree of abnormality of sural or peroneal nerve conduction did not have an effect on the frequency of MNW [61]. Stevens and colleagues [62] reviewed the medical records of 1016 patients diagnosed with carpal tunnel syndrome, and found that 56.8% of patients had a documented underlying condition associated with MNW, with a standardized morbidity ratio of 2.3 for DM. In the Rochester Diabetic Neuropathy cohort, electrophysiological evidence of median neuropathy at the wrist was found in 22% of type 1 DM and in 29% of type 2 DM patients without any symptoms. Clinical evidence for median neuropathy at the wrist was found in 9% of type 1 and 4% of type 2 diabetic patients. The mechanism for the increased risk for carpal tunnel syndrome in diabetics is unclear, and may relate to compression or to increased stiffness of connective tissue [58].

Diabetic radiculoplexus neuropathies

There are characteristic diabetic syndromes, which present subacutely with pain followed by weakness, that affect primarily patients with mild diabetes, called radiculoplexus neuropathies. Three main types can occur, alone or in combination, and include DCRPN, DTRN, and DLRPN. All forms (especially DLPRN) can be associated with weight loss.

Diabetic thoracic radiculopathy

Diabetic thoracic radiculopathies are a rare, but important complication of DM. These typically present with severe pain and dysesthesias along the trunk, chest, or abdominal wall, and often prompt extensive workups for underlying chest or abdominal pathology [63]. They can be symmetric and can involve multiple dermatomes [64]. They can be associated with weakness and outpouching of the abdominal wall, and can be mistaken for an abdominal hernia [65]. They can be associated with significant weight loss. They also can occur in patients who already have a significant distal symmetric polyneuropathy of the lower limbs or a DLRPN. EMG may show abnormalities of denervation in the thoracic paraspinal muscles or in abdominal muscles. The association of these with other forms of radiculoplexus neuropathies was noted by Bastron and Thomas [66] and termed diabetic polyradiculopathy. In case of uncertain diagnosis, the thermoregulatory sweat test can be useful, and may show pathologic loss of sweating in a thoracic or abdominal distribution. This sweat pattern has been found to correlate well with thoracic paraspinal muscle fibrillation potentials [67]. Skin biopsies in affected areas of the chest or trunk show a decrease in epidermal and dermal nerve fibers compared with biopsies from asymptomatic areas

[68]. Overall the prognosis is good; most patients reported in the literature have good recovery, usually within months to a year after the onset of their symptoms, without any specific treatment [65,69,70].

Diabetic lumbosacral radiculoplexus neuropathy

DLRPN occurs in approximately 1% of diabetic patients [7] and probably is the form of diabetic neuropathy that causes the most morbidity. It has been known variably by different names, including diabetic amyotrophy, Bruns-Garland syndrome, diabetic mononeuritis multiplex, diabetic polyradiculopathy, proximal diabetic neuropathy, and others. The authors prefer the designation of DLRPN, because it more accurately describes the extensive anatomic localization of the abnormalities in this disorder (ie, involvement of nerves at the root, plexus, and peripheral nerve levels). DLRPN more commonly affects patients with type 2 DM; the median age of presentation is 65 years, but the range in age is wide. These patients tend to have better glycemic control and a lower body mass index compared with a population-based study of diabetic patients (the Rochester Diabetic Neuropathy Study, RDNS) [71]. DLRPN patients also have a low rate of coexistent end-organ damage related to DM. In particular, cardiovascular disease and retinopathy occur at a significantly lower rate in these patients than in the diabetic population as a whole, suggesting an etiology other than metabolic derangement (longstanding hyperglycemic exposure) [71]. It is unclear what role DM plays in the pathophysiology of this disorder, as a very similar condition also is found in nondiabetic patients [72]. It seems likely that elevated blood sugars and DM is a risk factor for DLRPN but not the direct cause of it.

DLRPN usually presents with acute to subacute onset of severe lower extremity pain, either in the thigh or the leg, but ultimately spreading to the entire lower extremity. The presentation is usually unilateral or asymmetric and severe, and most patients will require narcotic pain medication for adequate control of their symptoms. The pain is of differing types and includes aching, burning, sharp stabbing, and contact allodynia [73]. Although pain is initially the worse symptom, weakness and atrophy become the main problem. Like the pain, the weakness usually begins focally but over time becomes widespread and bilateral. Weight loss is common; the median loss in the authors' series is 30 pounds. Numbness and tingling are also very common, and about 50% of patients have autonomic symptoms at the time of presentation, which can include orthostatic hypotension, genitourinary, and GI symptoms. Most patients eventually will have bilateral lower extremity signs and symptoms. In the authors' study of 33 prospectively evaluated patients who had DLRPN, only one did not develop bilateral symptomatology. These patients, however, may be more severely involved than the average patients who have DLRPN, because they were evaluated at a tertiary referral center. The mean time from onset to bilateral disease is 3 months. In the natural history of the disease, recovery is substantial but incomplete, and most patients have residual pain and some degree of leg weakness on long-term follow-up. Although one-half of the authors' patients required the use of a wheelchair, only three needed a wheelchair in long-term follow-up. Sixteen others, however, still required ongoing assistive aids (eg, walker, cane, brace) at long-term follow-up (2 years). Footdrop tended to be the biggest long-term problem as proximal segments reinnervated earlier and more completely [73].

Cerebrospinal fluid findings are suggestive of involvement of the root level, with elevated protein. The median value is 89 mg/dL, with a normal cell count being the typical pattern. This may suggest an inflammatory etiology, but it is not specific [73].

Neurophysiologic testing is most consistent with a process of primarily axonal degeneration. Nerve conduction studies show decreased peroneal and tibial compound muscle action potentials, and decreased sural sensory nerve action potentials, with significant side-to-side differences. The findings on needle electromyography implicate a multifocal process, which involves lumbosacral roots, plexus, and peripheral nerve. There is also objective evidence of autonomic neuropathy. In the authors' series, 14 DLRPN patients had autonomic testing performed, eight of whom had clinical autonomic symptoms. All 14 of these patients had abnormal composite autonomic severity scores (CASS), with 8 (57%) in the severely abnormal range. Of the four patients who had thermoregulatory sweat tests, all four were abnormal, with patchy anhidrosis of the affected areas of the lower limbs [73].

There is significant evidence to suggest that the primary pathologic process in DLRPN is ischemic injury from microvasculitis. As previously mentioned, the authors studied 33 prospectively evaluated cases with DLRPN who underwent distal cutaneous nerve biopsy (sural or superficial peroneal) [73]. The nerve pathology showed evidence of ischemic injury—focal or multifocal fiber degeneration and loss (Fig. 5), perineurial degeneration or thickening (Fig. 6), injury neuroma, and epineurial neovascularization (see Fig. 6). The ischemic injury seemed to be caused by altered immunity and microvasculitis. All nerves had increased inflammation; 15 of 33 had inflammatory cells in the vessel walls (suggestive of microvasculitis) (Fig. 7), and 19 of 33 had evidence of prior bleeding (hemosiderin) (see Fig. 6). In two cases, changes diagnostic of necrotizing vasculitis were seen [73]. The vasculitic changes tended to be those of microvasculitis involving microvessels and small venules with fragmentation of vessel walls and without fibrinoid necrosis.

Other authors also have noted these pathologic findings suggestive of a microvasculitic etiology for DLRPN. Llewelyn and colleagues [74] performed nerve biopsies (intermediate femoral cutaneous or sural) on 15 patients with findings consistent with DLRPN, and found inflammatory changes in five of these, four of which had microvasculitis and decreased numbers of myelinated fibers in all specimens. Kelkar and colleagues [75]

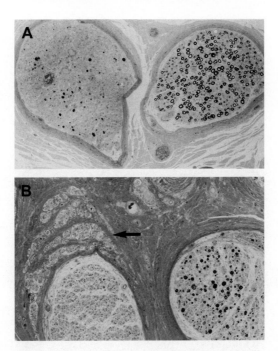

Fig. 5. Transverse epoxy sections (p-phenylenediamine) of distal sural nerves from patients with diabetic lumbosacral radiculoplexus neuropathy illustrating the dramatic focal fiber loss characteristic of the disorder (*A, fascicle on the left*) and the abortive microfascicular nerve regeneration (*B, as identified by the arrow*). Note that the abortive regeneration (injury neuroma) is made up of multiple regenerating fascicles and that they are situated adjacent to a fascicle devoid of myelinated fibers. Most of the fibers in the right fascicle in the lower panel are actively degenerating. As discussed in the text, these changes are indicative of ischemic injury that the authors attribute to a microscopic vasculitis. (*Reprinted from* Dyck PJB, Norell JE, Dyck PJ. Microvasculitis and ischemia in diabetic lumbosacral radiculoplexus neuropathy. Neurology 1999;53:2113–21; with permission.)

studied 15 patients with DLRPN by clinical, EMG, and laboratory evaluation, who had nerve and muscle biopsy. In four of these patients, there was inflammatory infiltration of vessel walls with PMNs and IgM deposits. In six of the patients, there was perivascular inflammation around epineurial blood vessels.

The findings of microvasculitis provide hope for effective treatment, particularly with immunomodulatory therapy. A retrospective study by Pascoe and colleagues [76] looked at the outcomes of patients with DLRPN either treated or untreated with immunosuppressive agents (either steroids, intravenous immune globulin, or plasma exchange). They found a higher rate of improvement (9 of 12 patients) in the treated group compared with the untreated group (17 of the 29 patients), although this was not statistically significant.

A randomized double-blinded placebo-controlled prospective treatment trial for DLRPN recently was completed by one of the authors [77].

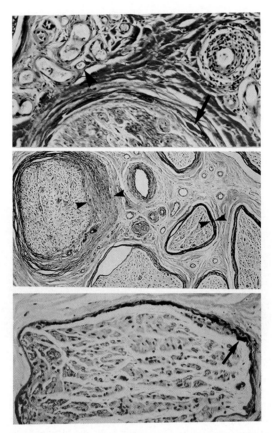

Fig. 6. Transverse paraffin sections of sural nerves showing changes seen in diabetic lumbosacral radiculoplexus neuropathy and non-diabetic lumbosacral radiculoplexus neuropathy. Upper panel, Masson's trichrome stain, showing inflammation in the wall of an epineurial microvessel (*right upper*), probably fibrinoid degeneration of the perineurium (*long arrow*), and a region of neovascularization (*arrowhead*). Middle panel, Luxol fast blue-periodic acid Schiff stain, showing several fascicles surrounded by normal thickness perineurium (*right middle, between the arrowheads*) and one fascicle with extremely thick perineurium (*left middle, between the arrowheads*). The authors attribute the latter finding to scarring and repair after ischemic injury (note all fascicles are devoid of myelinated fibers). Lower panel, Turnbull blue stain, showing accumulation of hemosiderin (*iron stains bright blue, arrow*) deposited along the inner aspects of the perineurium. All of these pathological features frequently are seen together and are explained best by ischemic injury. (*From* Dyck PJB, Windebank AJ. Diabetic and nondiabetic lumbosacral radiculoplexus neuropathies: new insights into pathophysiology and treatment. Muscle Nerve 2002;25:477–91; with permission. Copyright © 2002, Wiley Periodicals, Inc., A Wiley Company.)

Seventy-five patients with a mean age of 65.3 years were included in this trial, which randomized them to either placebo or intravenous methylprednisolone, starting at a dose of 1 g three times a week, with tapering over a 12-week period. Subjects had neuropathy impairment scores (NIS), and neuropathy impairment scores-lower limbs (NIS(LL)), as well as the

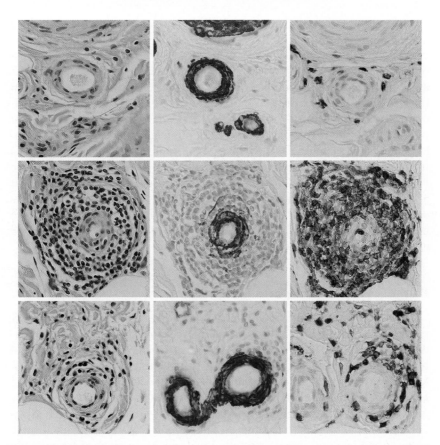

Fig. 7. Serial skip paraffin sections of a microvessel above (*upper panel*), at (*middle panel*), and below (*lower panel*) a region of microvasculitis in the sural nerve of a patient with diabetic lumbosacral radiculoplexus neuropathy. The sections on the left column are stained with hematoxylin and eosin; the sections in the middle column are reacted to antihuman smooth muscle actin (Dako), and the sections on the right column are reacted to leukocytes (CD 45). The smooth muscle of the tunica media in the region of microvasculitis (*middle panel*) is separated by mononuclear cells, fragmented and decreased in amount. The changes are those of a focal microvasculitis. (*Reprinted from* Sinnreich M, Taylor BV, Dyck PJB. Diabetic neuropathies classification, clinical features and pathophysiological basis. The Neurologist 2005;11(2): 63–79; with permission.)

neuropathy symptoms and change (NSC) taken at baseline, and at weeks 1, 6, 12, 24, 36, 52, and 104. The primary outcome measure for this study was time to improvement in NIS(LL) by four points. Both the steroid and the placebo group had significant improvement in the NIS and NIS(LL) by the end of the study. There was not a significant difference between the two groups in time to improvement in the NIS(LL) by four points, even though the treated group reached this endpoint over 30 days sooner. The patients treated with methylprednisolone, however, reported a significantly greater symptom improvement, particularly in regards to pain and positive neuropathic symptoms [77].

Although the primary outcome measure was not met for methylprednis-olone treatment of DLRPN, there was a statistically significant improvement in secondary endpoints of pain and positive sensory symptoms in the treated group over the placebo group, which is encouraging. As previously noted, the natural history of DLRPN is one of improvement of pain symptoms over time, and marked but often incomplete recovery of motor function. It is unclear if the lack of significant improvement in NIS(LL) in the steroid-treated group compared with the placebo group may have been related to timing of treatment. The study subjects were evaluated at a tertiary referral center, and so typically were not seen early in their disease course. It may be that, if prompt diagnosis and steroid treatment occurred early in the disease, it may have prevented some of the disease and have had a large impact on their neurological impairment.

Diabetic cervical radiculoplexus neuropathy

Although DLRPN is a much more familiar branch of the DRPN spectrum, the cervical segment also can be involved. In the authors' study of patients who had DLRPN, 3 out of 33 patients (10%) had coexistent bilateral but asymmetric cervical radiculoplexus neuropathies [73]. Katz and colleagues [78] reviewed medical records of 60 consecutive patients who had DLRPN and found that nine of them (15%) also had upper extremity involvement. The average age of these patients with cervicobrachial involvement was 59 years old, and all had type 2 DM. Four of these nine patients had bilateral upper extremity involvement. In eight of the nine patients, weakness was restricted to or most prominent in distal muscles, while only one patient had isolated proximal arm weakness. Only one patient was free of sensory loss, and most also had pain. All of these patients had electrodiagnostic testing, and seven had evaluation of an upper extremity; these showed evidence of denervation in affected muscles. Two of the patients were lost to follow-up, but the remaining seven had improvement in their arm symptoms and signs over a period of up to 9 months; three of those patients received treatment with some type of immunomodulatory regimen [78].

Summary

The spectrum of DM-associated neuropathies is large, and knowledge of these entities continues to evolve. There can be nerve damage from metabolic injury, compressive injury, ischemic injury, and from altered immunity, and these varied pathologies can present in many different ways. Identifying the pathogenesis of these entities is valuable, as there are clear differences in treatment strategies, which may range from lifestyle modification and strict glucose control to immunosuppressant medications, and can make significant impact in the quality of life of patients suffering from DM. To do this effectively, the caring physician needs to be able to make the correct diagnosis first, before starting the appropriate therapy.

References

[1] Leyden E. Beitrag zur Klinik des Diabetes mellitus. Wien Med Wochenschr 1893;43:926.
[2] Dyck PJB, Dyck PJ. Paresthesia, pain, and weakness in hands of diabetic patients is attributable to mononeuropathies or radiculopathy, not polyneuropathy: The Rochester (RDNS) and Pancreas Renal Transplant (MC-PRT) studies. Neurology 1998;50:A333.
[3] Tracy JA, Dyck PJB, Harper CM, et al. Hand symptomatology in diabetes usually due to mononeuropathy, not polyneuropathy. Ann Neurol 2005;58(Suppl 9):S36.
[4] Dyck PJ, O'Brien PC, Litchy WJ, et al. Monotonicity of nerve tests in diabetes. Subclinical nerve dysfunction precedes diagnosis of polyneuropathy. Diabetes Care 2005;28(9): 2192–200.
[5] Gregersen G. Diabetic neuropathy: influence of age, sex metabolic control, and duration of diabetes on motor conduction velocity. Neurology 1967;17:972–80.
[6] Dyck PJ, Davies JL, Wilson DM, et al. Risk factors for severity of diabetic polyneuropathy. Intensive longitudinal assessment of the Rochester Diabetic Neuropathy Study cohort. Diabetes Care 1999;22(9):1479–86.
[7] Dyck PJ, Kratz KM, Karnes JL, et al. The prevalence by staged severity of various types of diabetic neuropathy, retinopathy, and nephropathy in a population-based cohort: the Rochester Diabetic Neuropathy Study. Neurology 1993;43(4):817–24.
[8] Yasuda H, Dyck PJ. Abnormalities of endoneurial microvessels and sural nerve pathology in diabetic neuropathy. Neurology 1987;37:20–8.
[9] The Diabetes Control and Complications Trial Research Group. The effect of intensive diabetes therapy on the development and progression of neuropathy. Ann Intern Med 1995; 122(8):561–8.
[10] Nagamatsu M, Nickander KK, Schmelzer JD, et al. Lipoic acid improves nerve blood flow, reduces oxidative stress, and improves distal nerve conduction in experimental diabetic neuropathy. Diabetes Care 1995;18(8):1160–7.
[11] Ametov AS, Barinov A, Dyck PJ, et al. The sensory symptoms of diabetic polyneuropathy are improved with alpha-lipoic acid. The Sydney trial. Diabetes Care 2003;26(3):770–6.
[12] Ziegler D, Hanefeld M, Ruhnau KJ, et al. Treatment of symptomatic diabetic polyneuropathy with the antioxidant alpha-lipoic acid (ALADIN III study group). Diabetes Care 1999; 22(8):1296–301.
[13] Cameron NE, Eaton SE, Cotter MA, et al. Vascular factors and metabolic interactions in the pathogenesis of diabetic neuropathy. Diabetologia 2001;44(11):1973–88.
[14] Dyck PJ, Zimmerman BR, Vilen TH, et al. Nerve glucose, fructose, sorbitol, myo-inositol, and fiber degeneration and regeneration in diabetic neuropathy. N Engl J Med 1988;319(9): 542–8.
[15] Benstead TJ, Sangalang VE. Nerve microvessel changes in diabetes are prevented by aldose reductase inhibition. Can J Neurol Sci 1995;22(3):192–7.
[16] Judzewitsch RG, Jaspan JB, Polonsky KS, et al. Aldose reductase inhibition improves nerve conduction velocity in diabetic patients. N Engl J Med 1983;308(3):119–25.
[17] Fagius J, Brattberg A, Jameson S, et al. Limited benefit of treatment of diabetic polyneuropathy with an aldose reductase inhibitor: a 24-week controlled trial. Diabetologia 1985;28(6): 323–9.
[18] Boulton AJ, Levin S, Comstock J. A multicentre trial of the aldose reductase inhibitor, tolrestat, in patients with symptomatic diabetic neuropathy. Diabetologia 1990;33(7):431–7.

[19] Krentz AJ, Honigsberger L, Ellis SH, et al. A 12-month randomized controlled study of the aldose reductase inhibitor ponalrestat in patients with chronic symptomatic diabetic neuropathy. Diabet Med 1992;9(5):463–8.

[20] Apfel SC, Kessler JA, Adornato BT, et al. Recombinant human nerve growth factor in the treatment of diabetic polyneuropathy. Neurology 1998;51(3):695–702.

[21] McArthur JC, Yiannoutsos C, Simpson DM, et al. A phase II trial of nerve growth factor for sensory neuropathy associated with HIV infection. AIDS Clinical Trials Group Team 291. Neurology 2000;54(5):1080–8.

[22] Apfel SC, Schwartz S, Adornato BT, et al. Efficacy and safety of recombinant human nerve growth factor in patients with diabetic polyneuropathy. A randomized controlled trial. JAMA 2000;284:2215–21.

[23] Low PA, Benrud-Larson LM, Sletten DM, et al. Autonomic symptoms and diabetic neuropathy: a population-based study. Diabetes Care 2004;27(12):2942–7.

[24] Burgos LG, Ebert TJ, Asiddao C, et al. Increased intraoperative cardiovascular morbidity in diabetics with autonomic neuropathy. Anesthesiology 1989;70(4):591–7.

[25] Ewing DJ, Boland O, Neilson JM, et al. Autonomic neuropathy, QT interval lengthening, and unexpected deaths in male diabetic patients. Diabetologia 1991;34(3):182–5.

[26] Suarez GA, Clark VM, Norell JE, et al. Sudden cardiac death in diabetes mellitus: risk factors in the Rochester diabetic neuropathy study. J Neurol Neurosurg Psychiatry 2005;76(2): 240–5.

[27] Genuth S, Alberti KG, Bennett P, et al. Follow-up report on the diagnosis of diabetes mellitus. Diabetes Care 2003;26(11):3160–7.

[28] Center for Disease Control and Prevention. Prevalence of diabetes and impaired fasting glucose in adults—United States, 1999–2000. MMWR Morb Mortal Wkly Rep 2003;52(35):833–7.

[29] Harris MI, Flegal KM, Cowie CC, et al. Prevalence of diabetes, impaired fasting glucose, and impaired glucose tolerance in U.S. adults. The Third National Health and Nutrition Examination Survey, 1988–1994. Diabetes Care 1998;21(4):518–24.

[30] Harris MI, Eastman RC, Flegal KM, et al. Comparison of diabetes diagnostic categories in the United States population according to 1997 American Diabetes Association and 1985 World Health Organization diagnostic criteria. Diabetes Care 1997;20(12):1859–62.

[31] Singleton JR, Smith AG, Bromberg MB. Increased prevalence of impaired glucose tolerance in patients with painful sensory neuropathy. Diabetes Care 2001;24(8):1448–53.

[32] Sumner CJ, Sheth S, Griffin JW, et al. The spectrum of neuropathy in diabetes and impaired glucose tolerance. Neurology 2003;60(1):108–11.

[33] Hoffman-Snyder C, Smith BE, Ross MA, et al. Value of the oral glucose tolerance test in the evaluation of chronic idiopathic axonal polyneuropathy. Arch Neurol 2006;63(8): 1075–9.

[34] Thrainsdottir S, Malik RA, Dahlin LB, et al. Endoneurial capillary abnormalities presage deterioration of glucose tolerance and accompany peripheral neuropathy in man. Diabetes 2003;52(10):2615–22.

[35] Smith AG, Ramachandran P, Tripp S, et al. Epidermal nerve innervation in impaired glucose tolerance and diabetes-associated neuropathy. Neurology 2001;57(9):1701–4.

[36] Smith AG, Russell J, Feldman EL, et al. Lifestyle intervention for prediabetic neuropathy. Diabetes Care 2006;29(6):1294–9.

[37] Eriksson KF, Nilsson H, Lindgarde F, et al. Diabetes mellitus but not impaired glucose tolerance is associated with dysfunction in peripheral nerves. Diabet Med 1994;11(3):279–85.

[38] Hughes RA, Umapathi T, Gray IA, et al. A controlled investigation of the cause of chronic idiopathic axonal polyneuropathy. Brain 2004;127:1723–30.

[39] Rundles RW. Diabetic neuropathy: general review with report of 125 cases. Medicine (Baltimore) 1945;24:111–21.

[40] Ellenberg M. Diabetic neuropathic cachexia. Diabetes 1974;23(5):418–23.

[41] Archer AG, Watkins PJ, Thomas PK, et al. The natural history of acute painful neuropathy in diabetes mellitus. J Neurol Neurosurg Psychiatry 1983;46:491–9.

[42] Wilson JL, Sokol DK, Smith LH, et al. Acute painful neuropathy (insulin neuritis) in a boy following rapid glycemic control for type 1 diabetes mellitus. J Child Neurol 2003;18(5): 365–7.

[43] Llewelyn JG, Thomas PK, Fonseca V, et al. Acute painful diabetic neuropathy precipitated by strict glycaemic control. Acta Neuropathol (Berl) 1986;72(2):157–63.

[44] Kihara M, Zollman PJ, Smithson IL, et al. Hypoxic effect of exogenous insulin on normal and diabetic peripheral nerve. Am J Physiol 1994;266(6 Pt 1):E980–5.

[45] Tesfaye S, Malik R, Harris N, et al. Arterio-venous shunting and proliferating new vessels in acute painful neuropathy of rapid glycaemic control (insulin neuritis). Diabetologia 1996; 39(3):329–35.

[46] Jaspan JB, Wollman RL, Bernstein L, et al. Hypoglycemic peripheral neuropathy in association with insulinoma: implication of glucopenia rather than hyperinsulinism. Medicine (Baltimore) 1982;61:33–44.

[47] Westfall SG, Felten DL, Mandelbaum JA, et al. Degenerative neuropathy in insulin-treated diabetic rats. J Neurol Sci 1983;61(1):93–107.

[48] Sima AA, Zhang WX, Greene DA. Diabetic and hypoglycemic neuropathy—a comparison in the BB rat. Diabetes Res Clin Pract 1989;6(4):279–96.

[49] Guisado R, Arieff AI. Neurologic manifestations of diabetic comas: correlation with biochemical alterations in the brain. Metabolism 1975;24(5):665–79.

[50] Timperley WR, Preston FE, Ward JD. Cerebral intravascular coagulation in diabetic ketoacidosis. Lancet 1974;1(7864):952–6.

[51] Atkin SL, Coady AM, Horton D, et al. Multiple cerebral haematomata and peripheral nerve palsies associated with a case of juvenile diabetic ketoacidosis. Diabet Med 1995;12(3): 267–70.

[52] Bonfanti R, Bognetti E, Meschi F, et al. Disseminated intravascular coagulation and severe peripheral neuropathy complicating ketoacidosis in a newly diagnosed diabetic child. Acta Diabetol 1994;31(3):173–4.

[53] Krendel DA, Costigan DA, Hopkins LC. Successful treatment of neuropathies in patients with diabetes mellitus. Arch Neurol 1995;52(11):1053–61.

[54] Laughlin RS, Dyck PJ, Melton LJ, et al. The incidence and prevalence of chronic inflammatory demyelinating polyneuropathy in Olmsted County and the role of diabetes mellitus. Muscle Nerve 2006;34(4):512–3, S006.

[55] Gorson KC, Ropper AH, Adelman LS, et al. Influence of diabetes mellitus on chronic inflammatory demyelinating polyneuropathy. Muscle Nerve 2000;23(1):37–43.

[56] Stewart JD, McKelvey R, Durcan L, et al. Chronic inflammatory demyelinating polyneuropathy (CIDP) in diabetics. J Neurol Sci 1996;142(1–2):59–64.

[57] Watanabe K, Hagura R, Akanuma Y, et al. Characteristics of cranial nerve palsies in diabetic patients. Diabetes Res Clin Pract 1990;10(1):19–27.

[58] Dyck PJ, Giannini C. Pathologic alterations in the diabetic neuropathies of humans: a review. J Neuropathol Exp Neurol 1996;55(12):1181–93.

[59] Trigler L, Siatkowski RM, Oster AS, et al. Retinopathy in patients with diabetic ophthalmoplegia. Ophthalmology 2003;110(8):1545–50.

[60] Geoghegan JM, Clark DI, Bainbridge LC, et al. Risk factors in carpal tunnel syndrome. J Hand Surg [Br] 2004;29(4):315–20.

[61] Albers JW, Brown MB, Sima AA, et al. Frequency of median mononeuropathy in patients with mild diabetic neuropathy in the early diabetes intervention trial (EDIT). Tolrestat Study Group For Edit (Early Diabetes Intervention Trial). Muscle Nerve 1996;19(2): 140–6.

[62] Stevens JC, Beard CM, O'Fallon WM, et al. Conditions associated with carpal tunnel syndrome. Mayo Clin Proc 1992;67(6):541–8.

[63] Kikta DG, Breuer AC, Wilbourn AJ. Thoracic root pain in diabetes: the spectrum of clinical and electromyographic findings. Ann Neurol 1982;11(1):80–5.

[64] Waxman SG, Sabin TD. Diabetic truncal polyneuropathy. Arch Neurol 1981;38(1):46–7.

[65] Parry GJ, Floberg J. Diabetic truncal neuropathy presenting as abdominal hernia. Neurology 1989;39(11):1488–90.

[66] Bastron JA, Thomas JE. Diabetic polyradiculopathy: clinical and electromyographic findings in 105 patients. Mayo Clin Proc 1981;56:725–32.

[67] Fealey RD, Low PA, Thomas JE. Thermoregulatory sweating abnormalities in diabetes mellitus. Mayo Clin Proc 1989;64(6):617–28.

[68] Lauria G, McArthur JC, Hauer PE, et al. Neuropathological alterations in diabetic truncal neuropathy: evaluation by skin biopsy. J Neurol Neurosurg Psychiatry 1998;65(5):762–6.

[69] Chaudhuri KR, Wren DR, Werring D, et al. Unilateral abdominal muscle herniation with pain: a distinctive variant of diabetic radiculopathy. Diabet Med 1997;14(9):803–7.

[70] Longstreth GF. Diabetic thoracic polyradiculopathy: ten patients with abdominal pain. Am J Gastroenterol 1997;92(3):502–5.

[71] Dyck PJB, Windebank AJ. Diabetic and nondiabetic lumbosacral radiculoplexus neuropathies: new insights into pathophysiology and treatment. Muscle Nerve 2002;25(4):477–91.

[72] Dyck PJB, Norell JE, Dyck PJ. Nondiabetic lumbosacral radiculoplexus neuropathy. Natural history, outcome, and comparison with the diabetic variety. Brain 2001;124:1197–207.

[73] Dyck PJB, Norell JE, Dyck PJ. Microvasculitis and ischemia in diabetic lumbosacral radiculoplexus neuropathy. Neurology 1999;53:2113–21.

[74] Llewelyn JG, Thomas PK, King RHM. Epineurial microvasculitis in proximal diabetic neuropathy. J Neurol 1998;245(3):159–65.

[75] Kelkar PM, Masood M, Parry GJ. Distinctive pathologic findings in proximal diabetic neuropathy (diabetic amyotrophy). Neurology 2000;55(1):83–8.

[76] Pascoe MK, Low PA, Windebank AJ, et al. Subacute diabetic proximal neuropathy. Mayo Clin Proc 1997;72(12):1123–32.

[77] Dyck PJB, O'Brien P, Bosch EP, et al. The multicenter, double-blind controlled trial of IV methylprednisolone in diabetic lumbosacral radiculoplexus neuropathy. Neurology 2006; 66(5 Suppl 2):A191.

[78] Katz JS, Saperstein DS, Wolfe G, et al. Cervicobrachial involvement in diabetic radiculoplexopathy. Muscle Nerve 2001;24(6):794–8.

ELSEVIER
SAUNDERS

Phys Med Rehabil Clin N Am
19 (2008) 27–45

PHYSICAL MEDICINE
AND REHABILITATION
CLINICS OF
NORTH AMERICA

Neuromuscular Complications of Cancer and Cancer Treatments

Christian M. Custodio, MD[a,b,*]

[a]Department of Neurology, Rehabilitation Medicine Service, Memorial Sloan-Kettering
Cancer Center, 1275 York Avenue, Box 349, New York, NY 10065, USA
[b]Department of Rehabilitation Medicine, Joan and Sanford I. Weill Medical College
of Cornell University, 525 East 68th Street, New York, NY 10065, USA

Despite numerous advances in detection and treatment, cancer remains a major health problem in the United States. One in four deaths in the United States is caused by cancer, and cancer is the leading cause of death in individuals under 85 years of age [1]. However, death rates related to cancer have steadily decreased over the past few decades, and as a result, the number of survivors has exponentially increased. Increasingly, more and more secondary complications caused by cancer and its treatments are being recognized. Neuromuscular complications related to the underlying cancer itself, or caused by associated treatments, such as chemotherapy and radiation therapy, are common but are likely underreported. While neurologic involvement can occur in both the central and peripheral nervous systems at any level, this article focuses on the effects of cancer on the peripheral nervous system.

Using electrodiagnostic studies, neuromuscular abnormalities have been clinically detected in 2.5% to 5.5% of patients with lung or breast cancer, and in 28.5% of patients with various neoplasms [2]. Classification of these abnormalities can be organized either by etiology or by anatomic level. Many etiologies are possible. These include direct compression or infiltration, hematogenous spread, lymphatic spread, meningeal dissemination, or perineural spread. Peripheral nervous system involvement can also be caused by paraneoplastic syndromes, or from common secondary effects related to cancer, such as malnutrition, weight loss, or infection. Acquired neuropathies can result from side effects of the cancer treatments

* Department of Neurology, Rehabilitation Service, Memorial Sloan-Kettering Cancer Center, 1275 York Avenue, Box 349, New York, NY 10065.
E-mail address: custodc1@mskcc.org

1047-9651/08/$ - see front matter © 2008 Elsevier Inc. All rights reserved.
doi:10.1016/j.pmr.2007.10.001   *pmr.theclinics.com*

themselves, including surgery, chemotherapy, radiation therapy, hematopoietic stem cell transplantation, or immunologic therapy. Finally, patients may have pre-existing neurologic conditions, such as diabetic polyneuropathy, that can be exacerbated by cancer or its related treatments. Often, a combination of etiologies can be recognized in individual patients.

Involvement can occur at any level of the peripheral nervous system, including the anterior horn cells, nerve roots, sensory ganglia, brachial or lumbosacral plexus, single or multiple peripheral nerves, neuromuscular junction, and the muscle. Often multiple levels are involved. Neural damage at the cellular level may take place at the cell body, axon, myelin, or a combination of all of the above. The expected clinical findings are dependent on the location of the lesion.

Direct neuromuscular effects of cancer

Radiculopathy

A single or multilevel radiculopathy can result from primary or epidural metastatic tumor extension into the neural foramina (Fig. 1). All tumor types can metastasize to the spine, although the most common primary malignancies that do so include breast, lung, prostate, colon, thyroid, and kidney. Common primary malignant spinal tumors include multiple myeloma, plasmacytoma, and Ewing's and osteogenic sarcoma. After disc disease and spinal stenosis, tumors involving the spine and spinal cord are the most common causes of radiculopathy [3]. Although a degenerative etiology is more likely to cause symptoms, any patient with a history of cancer who presents with back pain and radicular symptoms and signs on

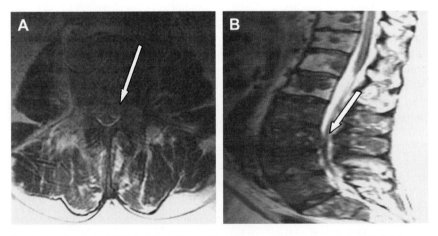

Fig. 1. Lumbar spine MRI demonstrating epidural disease with cauda equina and left L3 nerve root compression from metastatic prostate cancer (*arrows*). (*A*) T2 weighted axial image. (*B*) T2 weighted sagittal image.

physical examination warrants imaging, with magnetic resonance imaging (MRI) being the imaging modality of choice. An MRI of the total spine, not solely of the affected area, is subsequently obtained to determine extent of disease in instances where a neoplastic radiculopathy is identified.

Leptomeningeal metastases

Leptomeningeal disease is caused by metastatic involvement of the lepto-meninges from infiltrating cancer cells. The incidence of leptomeningeal me-tastasis ranges from 4% to 15% and is felt to be increasing [4]. The most common associated primary cancers are breast, lung, gastric, melanoma, and lymphomas [5]. Of the leukemias, leptomeningeal disease is most com-monly seen in acute lymphocytic leukemia [6]. Patients can present with an asymmetric array of symptoms resulting from polyradicular involvement, including focal and radicular pain, areflexia, paresthesias, and lower motor neuron weakness. There may be associated findings of nuchal rigidity, as well as upper motor neuron signs, especially if there is concomitant brain in-volvement. Cranial nerves are often involved as well, with the oculomotor, facial, and auditory nerves most commonly affected.

MRI with gadolinium of the spine and brain should be performed initially in all suspected cases. Nodular enhancement of the leptomeninges is almost pathognomonic (Fig. 2). The diagnosis is confirmed with the pres-ence of malignant cells on cerebrospinal fluid (CSF) cytology. However, there is a high initial false-negative rate on CSF studies of 40% to 50% [4]. Repeat CSF studies following an initial negative result improves the diagnostic yield to 90% [7]. Electrodiagnostic studies are consistent with a polyradiculopathy; however, underlying findings of an axonal, sensorimo-tor polyneuropathy, caused by prior chemotherapy treatment, can often be noted and can confuse the issue. Absent F-waves or prolonged F-wave latencies on nerve conduction studies are felt to be an early indicator of nerve root involvement, but are not specific for leptomeningeal disease [8]. Treatment is palliative and involves focal radiation therapy and chemother-apy, either intrathecal or systemic. Overall prognosis is poor and is depen-dent on multiple factors, including primary tumor type, extent of CSF disease as well as systemic disease, degree of neurologic deficit, and associ-ated medical comorbidities.

Plexopathy

Brachial plexopathies from neoplasms are usually the result of metastatic disease, with breast and lung being the most common primary sources [9]. In cancer patients, the frequency of neoplastic brachial plexopathy is 0.43% [10]. If a patient has a history of prior radiation therapy to the axillary or supraclavicular lymph nodes, secondary radiation-induced neoplasms, such as sarcomas, should also be considered. Symptoms include pain,

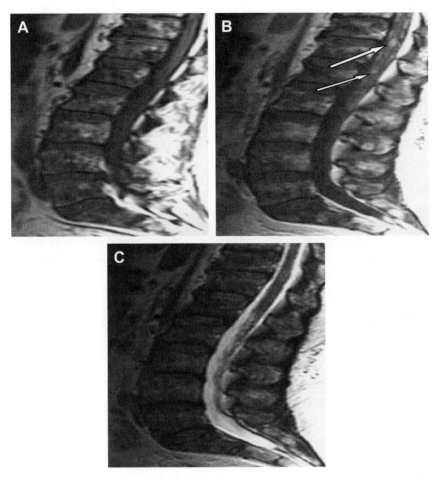

Fig. 2. Lumbar spine MRI demonstrating leptomeningeal metastasis from breast cancer. (*A*) T1 weighted sagittal image. (*B*) T1 weighted sagittal image postadministration of gadolinium. Note the nodular pattern of enhancement (*arrows*). (*C*) T2 weighted sagittal image.

paresthesias, numbness, and weakness in the distribution of plexus involvement. Metastases can involve any portion of the brachial plexus, but usually involve the lower trunk because of its proximity to axillary lymph nodes and the superior sulcus of the lung. Assessment of T1 fibers with needle electromyography is essential and can help guide further imaging studies [11]. The Pancoast syndrome is a distinct clinical presentation resulting from a superior pulmonary sulcus tumor, presenting with findings of a lower trunk brachial plexopathy and a unilateral Horner's syndrome [12]. MRI of the brachial plexus is usually diagnostic (Fig. 3).

Neoplastic lumbosacral plexopathies can result from metastatic disease, but are much more likely to be caused by direct extension of local tumor

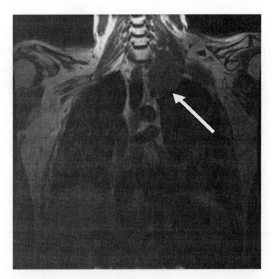

Fig. 3. Brachial plexus MRI demonstrating a superior pulmonary sulcus tumor (Pancoast lesion) (*arrow*).

or perineural spread [13]. Common tumors involved include colon, gynecologic tumors, lymphomas, and sarcomas. As in brachial plexopathies, neuropathic symptoms will be in the distribution of involvement, and MRI of the lumbosacral plexus is helpful in the diagnosis.

Neuropathy

Mononeuropathies most often result from the direct compression or invasion from tumor, such as an isolated radial neuropathy caused by a primary osteogenic sarcoma, or a bone metastasis involving the spiral groove of the humerus. Malignant nerve sheath tumors are rare and usually arise from plexiform neurofibromas [11]. There is a high association with neurofibromatosis type 1. The clinical presentation depends on the individual nerve involved, but severe pain and rapidly growing tumors suggest malignant transformation [14].

Diffuse peripheral nerve infiltration from cancer is rare but has been reported in hematologic malignancies, such as non-Hodgkin's lymphoma and chronic lymphocytic leukemia [15,16]. Amyloid deposition in primary amyloidosis and multiple myeloma can also result in diffuse polyneuropathy [17].

Myopathy

Focal myopathies from tumor involvement are rare, and usually result from direct infiltration from underlying bony metastases or local lymph node involvement, rather than from hematogenous spread. A more proximal myopathy, associated with macroglossia and muscle pseudohypertrophy, is an uncommon manifestation of primary amyloidosis. Muscle biopsy is diagnostic and demonstrates amyloid deposition surrounding muscle fibers and blood vessels. The selection of muscle to biopsy can be guided by electrodiagnostic findings. Needle electromyography demonstrates myopathic motor unit potentials or a mixture of large and small motor unit potentials, with fibrillation potentials noted primarily in proximal muscles [18].

Paraneoplastic syndromes

Neuromuscular paraneoplastic syndromes cause damage to the peripheral nervous system as a result of remote effects from a malignant neoplasm or its metastases [19]. Although rare, it is important to recognize these syndromes. The clinical presentation is usually more rapidly progressive and severe than what would normally be expected in a noncancerous etiology. They often precede the diagnosis of cancer, and early recognition may increase survival. Treatment of the underlying malignancy usually results in improvement of neurologic symptoms. In some disorders, neuronal antigens expressed by the tumor result in an autoimmune response against both the tumor as well as healthy neural tissue, and identification of these markers can help facilitate the diagnosis of a primary tumor. Although some syndromes are associated with an identifiable neuro-oncologic autoantibody, frequently no such marker is detected.

Almost all tumor types have been associated with paraneoplastic syndromes, and any part of the nervous system can be affected. There are, however, certain tumors that have a higher association with paraneoplastic syndromes, with neuroblastoma most often seen in children and small-cell lung cancer most often seen in adults. Paraneoplastic opsoclonus-myoclonus occurs in 2% to 3% of children with neuroblastoma. A small number (1%–3%) of patients with small-cell lung cancer develop Lambert-Eaton myasthenic syndrome (LEMS) or some other paraneoplastic syndrome [20].

Sensory neuronopathy

Paraneoplastic sensory neuronopathy or ganglionopathy presents with either an acute or insidious onset of pain and sensory loss. Clinical findings of sensory ataxia and pseudoathetosis are often present at various levels of severity. The findings can be diffuse but are commonly more severe in the upper extremities and may be asymmetric. Motor dysfunction is usually absent; however, sensory neuronopathy can sometimes be seen, along with a more diffuse paraneoplastic neurologic syndrome involving encephalomyelitis, autonomic neuropathy, and motor neuronopathy [19]. A pattern of more severe sensory abnormalities on nerve conduction studies in the upper extremities, compared with the lower extremities, helps distinguish this entity from a length-dependent sensory neuropathy. The most common associated neoplasm is small-cell lung cancer; however, breast, renal, chondrosarcoma, and lymphoma have also been implicated. The presence of anti-Hu antibodies helps support the diagnosis of paraneoplastic sensory neuronopathy.

Sensorimotor polyneuropathy

The diagnosis of a true paraneoplastic distal, symmetric, sensorimotor polyneuropathy is difficult to confirm, as there are many more likely known etiologies that can cause this pattern of involvement, including diabetes mellitus, nutritional deficiencies, and toxic exposure, such as chemotherapy. A subacute, sensorimotor polyneuropathy as a paraneoplastic syndrome is therefore a diagnosis of exclusion. Symptoms include pain, paresthesias, numbness, and weakness in a stocking-glove distribution, along with hyporeflexia. A more rapidly progressive course may be the only distinguishing factor differentiating a paraneoplastic syndrome from an idiopathic or diabetic etiology. Electrodiagnostic findings are consistent with an axonal process. This syndrome has been associated with lung and breast cancer [21].

Vasculitic neuropathy

A pattern of clinical and electrophysiologic involvement resembling mononeuritis multiplex may represent a paraneoplastic vasculitic neuropathy. This syndrome has been most commonly reported in association with small-cell lung cancer and lymphoma [22]. Further support for a vasculitis includes an elevated erythrocyte sedimentation rate, and an elevated cerebrospinal fluid protein level. The anti-Hu antibody has also been associated with this syndrome [23]. Biopsy of the sural nerve confirms microvascular involvement. In addition to treating any underlying malignancy, the neuropathic symptoms may also respond to immunosuppressive therapy directed against the vasculitis.

Lambert-Eaton myasthenic syndrome

LEMS is a presynaptic disorder of neuromuscular transmission, and is perhaps the best understood paraneoplastic neuromuscular syndrome. Clinically, patients present with fatigue, proximal weakness, hyporeflexia, and autonomic dysfunction. Repetitive strength testing may reveal a "warming-up" phenomenon, where one can display an initial increase in strength with repetition followed by eventual fatigue. Bulbar involvement is rare. LEMS tends to affect adults greater than 40 years of age, and has a male predominance. It can occur independent from cancer, but up to 40% to 60% of cases have been shown to be associated with small-cell lung cancer [9]. LEMS has also been reported to be associated with lymphoma, breast, ovarian, pancreatic, and renal malignancies.

Electrodiagnostic studies are invaluable in the diagnosis of LEMS. Motor responses are reduced in amplitude at baseline. Sensory responses are normal. Repetitive stimulation of motor nerves at low frequency (2 Hz–3 Hz) demonstrates a further decrement in amplitude. Following brief isometric exercise, facilitation occurs and compound muscle action potential amplitudes show at least a 100% increase [24]. This finding is almost pathognomonic for LEMS (see Fig. 3). Antibodies directed against the P/Q-type voltage-gated calcium channels are seen in up to 92% of LEMS patients [9]. Management involves administration of 3, 4 diaminopyridine and treatment of any underlying malignancy.

Myasthenia gravis

Myasthenia gravis (MG) is a postsynaptic disorder of neuromuscular transmission and its relationship with benign thymomas is widely recognized. MG occurs in 30% of patients with thymoma, and 15% of patients with MG are found to have thymoma on further radiographic evaluation [21]. Patients present with fatigue and proximal weakness, most notably in ocular and bulbar muscles. Electrodiagnostic studies demonstrate a decremental response in compound muscle potential amplitude with 2-Hz to 3-Hz repetitive stimulation. Unlike LEMS, baseline motor amplitudes are normal in MG, except in severe cases. Immediately following brief exercise, a repair of the decrement is noted. Postactivation exhaustion, with return of the decremental response, is noted 2 to 4 minutes after exercise. Patients under 60 years of age with generalized weakness, or patients with a documented thymoma, are treated via thymectomy [25]. Treatment can also involve the use of cholinesterase inhibitors or immunosuppressive agents.

Syndromes of neuromuscular hyperactivity

Hyperactivity syndromes, such as Stiff-person syndrome or neuromyotonia (Isaac's syndrome), are rare but have been associated with malignancies, including small-cell lung cancer, breast cancer, lymphoma, and invasive thymoma [26–28]. Stiff-person syndrome is a disorder characterized by muscle rigidity and a worsening of symptoms with exposure to certain triggers, such as loud noise or startle. Continuous motor unit activity is noted on needle electromyography, but otherwise electrodiagnostic findings are unremarkable. Antibodies to glutamic acid decarboxylase are present in up to 60% of patients; in some instances there is an association with antibodies against the presynaptic cell membrane protein amphiphysin. Isaac's syndrome is an autoimmune channelopathy that has been reported in association with Hodgkin's lymphoma as well as plasmacytoma [29,30]. Antibodies to voltage-gated potassium channels are present in 50% of patients. Continuous motor unit activity is again noted on needle EMG, however unlike Stiff-person syndrome, the symptoms and findings persist during sleep. Neurotonic discharges may also be present.

Myopathy

The findings of a symmetric, proximal myopathy on clinical examination and electrodiagnostic testing can also lead to the discovery of an undiagnosed cancer. Although their classification as a true paraneoplastic syndrome is controversial, polymyositis, and especially dermatomyositis, are associated with an increased incidence of malignancy compared with the general population [31]. Breast, lung, and gynecologic malignancies are most frequently implicated. Paraneoplastic necrotizing myopathy [32] and carcinoid myopathy are syndromes distinct from polymyositis or dermatomyositis. Carcinoid tumors may be associated with a progressive myopathy that has its onset years after the carcinoid syndrome [21].

Motor neuron disease

With regard to motor neuron disease syndromes, as mentioned previously the anti-Hu-associated paraneoplastic encephalomyelitis, sensory neuronopathy, and motor neuropathy syndrome has a strong link with small-cell lung cancer. Subacute motor neuropathy and primary lateral sclerosis have been associated with lymphoma and breast cancer, respectively [33]. There is no known association between cancer and amyotrophic lateral sclerosis; however, in newly diagnosed motor neuron disease a screening for cancer is usually part of the exclusionary diagnostic workup.

Neuropathy associated with plasma cell dyscrasias

Neuropathies associated with paraproteinemias and plasma cell dyscrasias warrant special consideration. Although not considered true paraneoplastic syndromes, there is a high association of neuropathies with these disorders and the presence of monoclonal proteins. These disorders include monoclonal gammopathy of unknown significance (MGUS), Waldenström's macroglobulinemia, cryoglobulinemia, multiple myeloma, osteosclerotic myeloma, primary amyloidosis, non-Hodgkin's lymphoma, and the chronic leukemias [34]. Even a diagnosis of MGUS should raise concern, as approximately 20% of these patients will at some point develop a malignant plasma cell disorder. A pattern of mononeuritis multiplex or distal symmetric polyneuropathy can be seen in lymphomas, myelomas, or leukemias, particularly chronic lymphocytic leukemia. Electrodiagnostic studies are usually consistent with an axonal process, although in the case of osteosclerotic myeloma and POEMS (polyneuropathy, organomegaly, endocrinopathy, M protein, skin changes) syndrome, findings of both axonal loss and multisegmental demyelination can be seen. The electrodiagnostic findings in POEMS syndrome can be similar to those seen in chronic, inflammatory demyelinating polyradiculoneuropathy [35]. The monoclonal gammopathy in these disorders can involve IgM, IgG, or IgA proteins, and there is some evidence to suggest that the type of paraproteinemia correlates to the clinical and electrophysiologic characteristics of the neuropathy [36].

Indirect neuromuscular effects of cancer

Immunocompromised patients are at risk for multiple infections, but with regards to the peripheral nervous system the main pathogen is herpes zoster varicella. Reactivation of herpes zoster, leading to shingles, has been reported to occur in up to 34% of leukemia patients [37], with resulting radicular pain and potential postherpetic neuralgia. Sepsis with multisystem organ failure is a serious complication of cancer and reason for intensive care admission, and in this setting critical illness polyneuropathy and critical illness myopathy are often diagnosed [38]. Other acute weakness syndromes, such as MG, LEMS, and steroid myopathies must be excluded.

Weight loss is a common symptom of malignancy, and there is a higher risk of compression neuropathy, especially the peroneal nerve at the level of the fibular head. This is because the nerve is no longer protected by soft tissue and is more easily compressed against bony structures. A history of habitual leg crossing is sometimes elicited. There may be additional predisposition to injury, given exposure to neurotoxic chemotherapy, to be discussed later in this article. In addition to complications associated with weight loss, malnutrition can be further associated with a neuropathy, secondary to vitamin B_{12} deficiency. Renal failure from myeloma or amyloid involvement can result in a uremic neuropathy. Cachexia and related metabolic proximal myopathies affecting primarily type 2 muscle fibers are also seen.

Neuromuscular complications of cancer treatments

Surgery

Although uncommon, damage to the peripheral nervous system during the perioperative period can occur in both the cancer and noncancer patient. Because the nature of surgical procedures for the cancer patient is likely to be more complex, it is felt that the likelihood of complications is greater. There are no studies, however, comparing the incidence of unintentional nerve injury in the cancer surgery population to that in the general population. In addition, peripheral nerves are sometimes intentionally sacrificed in the cancer surgery patient to obtain local disease control. The pattern and extent of neurologic involvement following surgery depends on the location of the tumor, patient positioning during surgery, and the patient's overall preoperative status and propensity to nerve injury [39]. For example, through mechanisms mentioned previously, a cancer patient having undergone a significant amount of weight loss before treatment may be more susceptible to a perioperative peroneal neuropathy at the fibular head, resulting from positioning following a prolonged surgery and postoperative recovery period.

Perioperative neurapraxic injuries, resulting from compression of peripheral nerves, are well-recognized phenomena. It is felt that these injuries result from the patient's position during anesthesia or during the immediate post-surgical recovery period [40]. Common sites of injury and associated surgical procedures include brachial plexus injury during thoracotomy or mastectomy, given the abducted position of the involved upper extremity. Abduction of the upper extremity greater than 90 degrees during anesthesia will cause the humeral head to sublux inferiorly, resulting in compression and traction of the brachial plexus. Upon awakening, patients report varying degrees of pain, weakness, and numbness in both the upper and lower trunk distribution. Complete, spontaneous recovery within weeks is common, even in cases of severe plegia. Ulnar neuropathies at the elbow, resulting from arm boards used to secure intravenous lines, and radial neuropathies at the spiral groove, resulting from prolonged time in the lateral decubitus position, are also noted following thoracic surgery.

Compression of the femoral nerve or lumbar plexus can result from traction during pelvic surgery. Patients undergoing hip arthroplasty or acetabular reconstruction are prone to injury, with the peroneal division of the sciatic nerve being the most commonly affected nerve. Injuries to the superior gluteal, obturator, and femoral nerves have also been reported [41]. Cadaveric studies demonstrate that the lithotomy position, with the lower limbs placed in greater than 30 degrees of abduction, causes excessive traction on the obturator nerve. This strain is relieved, however, with concomitant hip flexion [42]. Finally, delayed postoperative hemorrhages and hematomas should be excluded in all patients who develop new neuropathic symptoms 24 to 48 hours after surgery.

There are a few specific neurotmetic surgical injuries that warrant consideration. The spinal accessory nerve is often sacrificed during radical or modified radical neck dissection for head and neck cancers. The branch to the trapezius is usually more affected than the branch innervating the sternocleidomastoid. A resulting drooped shoulder and lateral scapular winging can lead to chronic shoulder pain. During radical or modified radical mastectomy, the intercostal-brachial nerve is frequently damaged, resulting in pain and paresthesias involving the lateral chest wall and medial upper arm, predisposing patients to secondary adhesive capsulitis. Postthoracotomy pain syndrome is caused by sacrifice of the intercostal nerves, may have its onset weeks after surgery, and can persist for years. If there is new pain in the area of surgery, it is important to rule out tumor recurrence invading the chest wall, or thoracic vertebral body metastases causing compressive radiculopathy, before making a diagnosis of delayed postthoracotomy pain syndrome. Damage to lower extremity nerves is uncommon during abdominal or pelvic surgery, unless a tumor has already infiltrated nervous system structures. The rates of unintentional or planned nerve sacrifice are high in limb-sparing procedures for extremity sarcomas because of the need to achieve adequate tumor-free surgical margins. Electrodiagnostic studies performed immediately after surgery, and 2 to 3 weeks afterward, can help prognosticate neurologic recovery [43]. A thorough discussion of pain syndromes following amputation, including residual limb pain and phantom pain, is beyond the scope of this article.

Chemotherapy

Peripheral neuropathy is a common adverse effect of medications in general; however, when these medicines are used to treat life-threatening illnesses, such as cancer, it becomes challenging to balance the potentially functionally limiting side effects with the obvious benefits of chemotherapy. Side effects tend to be dose-dependent, although it is important to recognize pre-existing subclinical neuropathies or a family history of neuropathy, such as in the case of the hereditary sensory and motor neuropathies. The neurotoxic effects of chemotherapy in these patients can occur earlier than expected in the treatment course, and symptoms can be devastating and disabling [44–46]. Although almost all agents have been associated with neuropathies, there are a select number of chemotherapeutics that are especially prone to causing neuropathy. Chemotherapy induced neuropathy generally is characterized by axonal loss via Wallerian degeneration, and presents with a subacute, length-dependent, sensory greater than motor, polyneuropathy. The prognosis for neurologic recovery upon discontinuation of the offending agent is generally favorable, but depends on the severity of symptoms.

Two classes of chemotherapeutic agents in prevalent use are the vinca alkaloids and the taxanes. The vinca alkaloids—such as vincristine, vinblastine, and vinorelbine—are used in the treatment of solid tumors, lymphomas, and leukemias. They are usually given in combination with other chemotherapeutic agents. The mechanism of action with the vinca alkaloids is to arrest dividing cells in metaphase by binding tubulin and preventing its polymerization into microtubules. This is also the proposed mechanism of inducing neuropathy, by inhibiting anterograde and retrograde transport and causing axonal degeneration. Clinical features are those of a distal, symmetric, sensorimotor axonal polyneuropathy, affecting both large and small fibers. Taxanes, such as paclitaxel and docetaxel, are also used to treat solid tumors, such as breast and ovarian cancer. As in the vinca alkaloids, the taxane-induced neuropathy is a length-dependent sensorimotor polyneuropathy resulting from damage to the axonal microtubule system [47]. Similar agents, generally resulting in a length-dependent, axonal neuropathy affecting sensory greater than motor fibers, include thalidomide and bortezomib, both used in the treatment of multiple myeloma.

Etoposide is a lesser used agent but is useful in the treatment of lymphoma, leukemia, small-cell lung cancer, and testicular cancer. As in most drug-induced neuropathies, etoposide is associated with an axonal, distal, symmetric sensorimotor polyneuropathy. In addition, there have also been reports of an associated severe autonomic neuropathy with orthostatic hypotension and gastroparesis [9].

Platinum based compounds are used in the treatment of solid tumors, such as ovarian, testicular, and bladder cancer. They include agents such as cisplatin, carboplatin, and oxaliplatin. While platinum toxicity can also result in a distal, symmetric, sensorimotor polyneuropathy, there also appears to be preferential damage to the dorsal root ganglia, causing a sensory neuronopathy with clinical features, including sensory ataxia, and upper extremities being more affected than the lower extremities. A "coasting phenomenon" may be noted, where symptoms can progress for months following discontinuation of the platinum compound. Prognosis for recovery in a sensory ganglionopathy is poor.

Cytarabine is used in the treatment of hematologic cancers. There have been reports of severe sensorimotor polyneuropathy, resembling Guillain-Barré syndrome, with high dose administration of cytarabine [48]. Electrophysiologic studies demonstrate a mixed axonal and multifocal demyelinating process.

Hand-foot syndrome is an unusual complication of several chemotherapeutic agents, including 5-flurouracil, capecitabine, doxorubicin, docetaxel, and cytarabine. Clinical features include painful desquamation and discoloration of the palms and soles of the hands and feet. The pain is frequently described as burning in character. Clinical findings include reduced pain and temperature sensation, with preserved reflexes, proprioception, and strength. Electrodiagnostic studies are usually normal. Intraepidermal nerve fiber density evaluation demonstrates decreased numbers of small fibers, both proximally and distally, suggestive of a painful small fiber neuropathy [49].

Glucocorticosteroids are perhaps the most frequently used medications in the oncology patient. The primary use of corticosteroids in cancer patients is to control brain and spinal cord edema, but they are also used in the treatment of cancers, such as lymphoma. They are also helpful in treating pain, improving appetite, and managing nausea and vomiting caused by other chemotherapeutic agents. The major neuromuscular complication associated with corticosteroid use is steroid-induced myopathy. Patients present clinically, with proximal weakness and myalgias and without sensory abnormalities. Muscle biopsies demonstrate type 2 muscle fiber atrophy. Needle electromyographic findings are unremarkable. Prolonged, high dose use of corticosteroids can cause steroid-induced diabetes, which can lead to all of the associated secondary complications of diabetes, including peripheral neuropathy.

Radiation therapy

Approximately 50% of all cancer patients will undergo radiation therapy at some point during the course of their disease, and radiation therapy is involved in approximately one quarter of all cancer cures [50]. As patients are living longer following cancer treatments, physicians are becoming more aware of late neuromuscular complications of therapy, especially radiation therapy. Side effects are essentially related to the dose of radiation and the volume of normal tissue that receives radiation [51]. Despite numerous advances with dose-fractionation schedules, beam conformation technology, and the advent of intensity modulated or image guided radiation therapy, it is still necessary to include normal tissue within the treatment field, much like a successful surgery requires adequate negative margins to achieve local disease control.

Radiation causes tissue injury primarily by the induction of apoptosis, a result of free radical-mediated DNA damage. Rapidly dividing cells, such as neoplastic cells, are particularly susceptible. Normal cells are also affected but to a lesser extent. In addition, radiation causes direct and indirect tissue injury that is mediated by a combination of chemokines, cytokines, and other growth factors. This includes activation of the coagulation system, inflammation, epithelial regeneration, and tissue remodeling. Although the exact pathophysiologic mechanism is not entirely understood, it is felt that this damage to the vascular endothelial system, causing abnormal collagen deposition and fibrosis in the perivascular and extracellular matrix, is the primary method resulting in damage to the underlying neuromuscular structures [50].

The clinical effects of radiation on peripheral nerves have been well documented. Any structure in the nervous system, both centrally and peripherally, is susceptible to radiation toxicity, including brain, spinal cord, and the nerve roots. However, the majority of studies and articles examining the phenomenon of radiation-induced damage to the peripheral nervous systems focus on radiation-induced plexopathy, specifically brachial plexopathy.

The primary differential diagnostic concern in a cancer patient with brachial plexopathy is distinguishing between a neoplastic and radiation-induced etiology. Occasionally, the two conditions can coexist. Classically, radiation-induced plexopathy is delayed in onset, pain is less common than in neoplastic plexopathy, and symptoms of weakness and paresthesias are usually progressive [52,53]. There is also more likely to be associated lymphedema in the involved limb. It has been reported that neoplastic plexopathy tends to preferentially affect the lower trunk, and radiation plexopathy the upper portion of the plexus; however, further studies suggest that plexus involvement may be more diffuse and with more overlap in both etiologies than previously suspected [54]. The presence of myokymic discharges and fasciculation potentials strongly suggests a radiation-induced contribution to plexus injury [53]. However, the absence of myokymic discharges does not exclude radiation damage. Even in the setting of classic EMG findings, follow-up imaging of the brachial plexus with MRI is indicated to exclude a concomitant compressive or infiltrating lesion, which could be caused by local recurrence, new metastases, or radiation-induced secondary tumors, such as sarcomas.

Originally thought to be relatively radioresistant, it is becoming more apparent that skeletal muscle is also susceptible to late onset effects of radiation therapy. The direct effect of radiation on muscle results in fibrosis and contracture [55]. There have been multiple reports of a late dropped head syndrome in patients who have received mantle field radiation therapy in the distant past as part of their treatment for Hodgkin's lymphoma [56,57]. Clinical features include slowly progressive atrophy of neck and shoulder girdle musculature. Neck flexor and extensor muscles are markedly weak, with remarkably preserved motor function in the shoulder girdle and upper extremities. Affected muscles have a firm, fibrotic character on palpation. The head tends to be in a forward-flexed position, with a secondary kyphotic spinal posture caused by anterior cervical muscle contracture. Secondary musculoskeletal complications related to impaired posture, such as rotator cuff impingement syndromes, are seen. Needle electromyography demonstrates low amplitude, short duration, polyphasic motor unit potentials in affected muscles, with normal or decreased insertional activity and rare, if any, fibrillation potentials. There may additionally be findings of a concomitant brachial plexopathy [58]. Creatinine kinase levels and inflammatory markers are normal. Muscle biopsy in one patient demonstrated nemaline rod depositions in affected muscles, while biopsy results from unaffected muscles was normal [56].

Trismus is a special myopathic condition where the muscles of mastication, especially the masseter and pterygoids, are affected by radiation therapy used in the treatment of head and neck cancers [59]. Patients present with contractures of affected muscles, with progressive loss of interincisal opening. Pain may or may not be present. Jaw contractures can create difficulties with eating, and malnutrition complications may occur. Oral hygiene is also compromised, which can also be complicated by xerostomia, another common side effect of radiation therapy.

The incidence of radiation-induced secondary tumors is directly proportional to the radiation dose, and inversely proportional to the patient age at which the radiation is administered [60]. Distinguishing between local recurrence, primary metastases, and new tumor types has obvious implications in prognosis and treatment options. Their neuromuscular effects, like other tumors, are dependent on their location in proximity to the peripheral nervous system, and could also result in indirect neurologic effects and associated paraneoplastic syndromes. Secondary tumors include bone and soft tissue sarcomas, leukemias, melanomas, and thyroid cancers.

Hematopoietic stem cell transplant

Hematopoietic stem cell transplantation is performed as part of the treatment for hematologic malignancies, such as leukemias, lymphomas, and multiple myeloma, as well as for select solid tumors and nonmalignant diseases. These patients will frequently receive additional chemotherapy or radiation therapy as part of their treatment regimen, and are susceptible to related neurotoxic effects, as described earlier. Common neurotoxic chemotherapeutic agents used in the setting of stem cell transplantation include cisplatin, paclitaxel, docetaxel, etoposide, thalidomide, and cytarabine. The chronic immunosuppressed state of these patients also makes them more prone to opportunistic infections and secondary peripheral neuropathies, such as herpes varicella zoster. Metabolic derangements, such as steroid-induced diabetes and malabsorption syndromes, are also common following transplantation, and can likewise result in secondary peripheral nervous system dysfunction.

Chronic graft-versus-host disease (GVHD) is the primary late-term complication associated with transplant. The graft, containing immunologically competent cells, reacts to host tissue antigens and performs an autoimmune response against the transplant recipient. Forty percent of patients having survived more than 100 days after transplant will develop GVHD [61]. There is a high association with chronic GVHD and autoimmune neuromuscular disorders, including inflammatory myopathies, myasthenia gravis, and both acute and chronic polyneuropathies.

Polymyositis, and to a lesser degree, dermatomyositis, are well recognized but uncommon complications of chronic GVHD. The incidence of polymyositis in the GVHD population is greater than that of the general population [62]. The clinical presentation, electrodiagnostic findings, and pathologic findings in GVHD-associated polymyositis are identical to idiopathic polymyositis. Differentiating an inflammatory myopathy from a steroid-induced myopathy is of obvious clinical importance.

MG in the setting of chronic GVHD usually develops between 2 and 5 years after transplantation, during tapering of immunosuppressive drug therapy [63]. Clinically and electrophysiologically, the findings are similar to typical autoimmune MG. Treatment regimens are likewise similar with equal efficacy. Acetylcholine receptor antibodies may or may not be present. There has not been a reported association with thymoma in patients with GVHD-associated MG.

Autoimmune neuropathies have also been associated with GVHD, and can present as either a distal symmetric sensorimotor polyneuropathy with characteristic electrodiagnostic findings, or as a syndrome with features similar to Guillain-Barré syndrome [64,65].

Summary

With numerous advancements in early detection and multimodal therapy, cancer has become a chronic disease. As the number of cancer survivors continue to increase, physiatrists and other neuromuscular disease specialists are more likely to encounter individuals with residual impairments, disabilities, or handicaps resulting from cancer or related treatments. The cancer patient is especially prone to injury directed at the peripheral nervous system at multiple levels. Tumors can directly compress or infiltrate vital nervous system structures, or can cause severe neuromuscular disorders through a paraneoplastic process. Immunocompromised cancer patients are susceptible to indirect neurologic insult through secondary mechanisms, such as infection or metabolic disorders. Cancer treatments themselves, including surgery, chemotherapy, radiation therapy, and hematopoietic stem cell transplant, can result in devastating neuromuscular complications. Recognition of associated neuromuscular complications of cancer and cancer treatments can be challenging because of the wide, multifactorial array of potential etiologies, but recognizing them is important in designing specific, individualized rehabilitation treatments to the oncologic patient and survivor.

References

[1] Jemal A, Siegel R, Ward E, et al. Cancer Statistics, 2007. CA Cancer J Clin 2007;57:43–66.
[2] Hughes R, Sharrack B, Rubens R. Carcinoma and the peripheral nervous system. J Neurol 1996;243:371–6.
[3] Shelerud RA, Paynter KS. Rarer causes of radiculopathy: spinal tumors, infections, and other unusual causes. Phys Med Rehabil Clin N Am 2002;13:646–96.
[4] Taillibert S, Laigle-Donadey F, Chodkiewicz C, et al. Leptomeningeal metastases from solid malignancy: a review. J Neurooncol 2005;75:85–99.
[5] Stubgen JP. Neuromuscular disorders in systemic malignancy and its treatment. Muscle Nerve 1995;18:636–48.
[6] Demopoulous A, DeAngelis LM. Neurologic complications of leukemia. Curr Opin Neurol 2002;15:691–9.
[7] Wasserstrom WR, Glass P, Posner JB. Diagnosis and treatment of leptomeningeal metastasis from solid tumors: experience with 90 patients. Cancer 1982;49:759–72.
[8] Argov Z, Siegal T. Leptomeningeal metastases: peripheral nerve and root involvement—clinical and electrophysiologic study. Ann Neurol 1985;17:593–6.
[9] Breimberg HR, Amato AA. Neuromuscular complications of cancer. Neurol Clin 2003;21:141–65.
[10] Jaeckle KA. Neurological manifestations of neoplastic and radiation-induced plexopathies. Semin Neurol 2004;24:385–93.
[11] Ferrante MA. Brachial plexopathies: classification, causes, and consequences. Muscle Nerve 2004;30:547–68.
[12] Pancoast HK. Superior pulmonary sulcus tumor. JAMA 1932;99:1391–6.
[13] Ladha SS, Spinner RJ, Suarez GA, et al. Neoplastic lumbosacral radiculoplexopathy in prostate cancer by direct perineural spread: an unusual entity. Muscle Nerve 2006;34:659–65.
[14] Antoine JC, Camdessanche JP. Peripheral nervous system involvement in patients with cancer. Lancet Neurol 2007;6:75–86.
[15] Kelly JJ, Karcher DS. Lymphoma and peripheral neuropathy: a clinical review. Muscle Nerve 2005;31:301–13.
[16] Amato AA, Dumitru D. Acquired neuropathies. In: Dumitru D, Amato AA, Zwarts MD, editors. Electrodiagnostic Medicine. 2nd edition. Philadelphia: Hanley and Blefus; 2002. p. 937–1041.

[17] Kelly JJ, Kyle RA, Miles JM, et al. The spectrum of peripheral neuropathy in myeloma. Neurology 1981;31:24–31.

[18] Rubin DI, Hermann RC. Electrophysiologic findings in amyloid myopathy. Muscle Nerve 1999;22:355–9.

[19] Darnell RB, Posner JB. Paraneoplastic syndromes involving the nervous system. N Engl J Med 2003;349:1543–54.

[20] Dropcho EJ. Neurologic paraneoplastic syndromes. Curr Oncol Rep 2004;6:26–31.

[21] Posner JB. Paraneoplastic syndromes. In: Posner JB, editor. Neurologic complications of cancer. 1st edition. Philadelphia: F.A. Davis; 1995. p. 353–85.

[22] Oh SJ. Paraneoplastic vasculitis of the peripheral nervous system. Neurol Clin 1997;15: 849–63.

[23] Younger D, Dalmau J, Inghirami G, et al. Anti-Hu-associated peripheral nerve and muscle microvasculitis. Neurology 1994;44:181–3.

[24] Stubblefield MD, Custodio CM, Franklin DJ. Cardiopulmonary rehabilitation and cancer rehabilitation. 3. Cancer rehabilitation. Arch Phys Med Rehabil 2006;87(3 Suppl 1): S65–71.

[25] Keesey JC. Clinical evaluation and management of myasthenia gravis. Muscle Nerve 2004; 29:484–505.

[26] Bateman DE, Weller RD, Kennedy P. Stiffman syndrome: a rare paraneoplastic disorder? J Neurol Neurosurg Psychiatry 1995;53:695–6.

[27] Rosin L, DeCamilli P, Butler M, et al. Stiff-man syndrome in a woman with breast cancer: an uncommon central nervous system paraneoplastic syndrome. Neurology 1998;50:84–8.

[28] Hagiwara H, Enomoto-Nakatani S, Sakai K, et al. Stiff-person syndrome associated with invasive thymoma: a case report. J Neurol Sci 2001;193:59–62.

[29] Caress JB, Abend WK, Preston DC, et al. A case of Hodgkin's lymphoma producing neuro-myotonia. Neurology 1997;49:258–9.

[30] Zifko U, Drlicek M, Machacek E, et al. Syndrome of continuous muscle fiber activity and plasmacytoma with IgM paraproteinemia. Neurology 1994;44:560–1.

[31] Yazici Y, Kagen LJ. The association of malignancy with myositis. Curr Opin Rheumatol 2000;12:498–500.

[32] Levin MI, Mozaffar T, Taher Al-Lozi M, et al. Paraneoplastic necrotizing myopathy: clinical and pathologic features. Neurology 1998;50:764–7.

[33] Younger DS. Motor neuron disease and malignancy. Muscle Nerve 2000;23:658–60.

[34] Ropper AH, Gorson KC. Neuropathies associated with paraproteinemias. N Engl J Med 1998;338:1601–7.

[35] Sung J, Kuwabara S, Ogawara K, et al. Patterns of nerve conduction abnormalities in POEMS syndrome. Muscle Nerve 2002;26:189–93.

[36] Suarez GA, Kelly JJ. Polyneuropathy associated with monoclonal gammopathy of undeter-mined significance: further evidence that IgM-MGUS neuropathies are different than IgG-MGUS. Neurology 1993;43:1304–8.

[37] Poulsen A, Schmiegelow K, Yssing M. Varicella zoster infections in children with acute lym-phoblastic leukemia. Pediatr Hematol Oncol 1996;13:231–8.

[38] Sliwa JA. Acute weakness syndromes in the critically ill patient. Arch Phys Med Rehabil 2000;81(3 Suppl):S45–52.

[39] Posner JB. Neurotoxicity of surgical and diagnostic procedures. In: Posner JB, editor. Neu-rologic Complications of Cancer. 1st edition. Philadelphia: F.A. Davis; 1995. p. 338–52.

[40] Dawson DM, Krarup C. Perioperative nerve lesions. Arch Neurol 1989;46:1355–60.

[41] DeHart MM, Riley LH Jr. Nerve injuries in total hip arthroplasty. J Am Acad Orthop Surg 1999;7:101–11.

[42] Litwiller JP, Wells RE Jr, Halliwill JR, et al. Effect on lithotomy positions on strain of the obturator and lateral femoral cutaneous nerves. Clin Anat 2004;17:45–9.

[43] Custodio CM. Barriers to rehabilitation of patients with extremity sarcomas. J Surg Oncol 2007;95:393–9.

[44] Graf WD, Chance PF, Lensch MW, et al. Severe vincristine neuropathy in Charcot-Marie-Tooth disease type 1A. Cancer 1996;77:1356–62.

[45] Chauvenet AR, Shashi V, Selsky C, et al. Vincristine-induced neuropathy as the initial presentation of Charcot-Marie-Tooth disease in acute lymphoblastic leukemia: a Pediatric Oncology Group study. J Pediatr Hematol Oncol 2003;25:316–20.

[46] Chaudhry V, Chaudhry M, Crawford TO, et al. Toxic neuropathy in patients with pre-existing neuropathy. Neurology 2003;60:337–40.

[47] Peltier AC, Russell JW. Recent advances in drug-induced neuropathies. Curr Opin Neurol 2002;15:633–8.

[48] Openshaw H, Slatkin NE, Stein AS, et al. Acute polyneuropathy after high-dose cytosine arabinoside in patients with leukemia. Cancer 1996;78:1899–905.

[49] Stubblefield MS, Custodio CM, Kaufmann P, et al. Small-fiber neuropathy associated with capecitabine (Xeloda)-induced hand-foot syndrome: a case report. Journal of Clinical Neuromuscular Disease 2006;7:128–32.

[50] Hauer-Jensen M, Fink LM, Wang J. Radiation injury and the protein C pathway. Crit Care Med 2004;32(5 Suppl):S325–30.

[51] Pan CC, Hayman JA. Recent advances in radiation oncology. J Neuroophthalmol 2004;24:251–7.

[52] Kori SH, Foley KM, Posner JB. Brachial plexus lesions in patients with cancer: 100 cases. Neurology 1981;31:45–50.

[53] Harper CM, Thomas JE, Cascino TL, et al. Distinction between neoplastic and radiation-induced brachial plexopathy, with emphasis on the role of EMG. Neurology 1989;39:502–6.

[54] Boyaciyan A, Oge AE, Yazici J, et al. Electrophysiological findings in patients who received radiation therapy over the brachial plexus: a magnetic stimulation study. Electroencephalogr Clin Neurophysiol 1996;101:483–90.

[55] Vissink A, Jansma J, Spijkervet FK, et al. Oral sequelae of head and neck radiotherapy. Crit Rev Oral Biol Med 2003;14:199–212.

[56] Portlock CS, Boland P, Hays AP, et al. Nemaline myopathy: a possible late complication of Hodgkin's disease therapy. Hum Pathol 2003;34:816–8.

[57] Rowin J, Cheng G, Lewis SL, et al. Late appearance of dropped head syndrome after radio-therapy for Hodgkin's disease. Muscle Nerve 2006;34:666–9.

[58] Okereke LI, Custodio CM, Stubblefield MD. Bilateral lower-trunk brachial plexopathy and proximal myopathy 19 years after mantle field radiation for Hodgkin's disease: a case report. Arch Phys Med Rehabil 2004;85:e23–4.

[59] Sciubba JJ, Goldenberg D. Oral complications of radiotherapy. Lancet Oncol 2006;7:175–83.

[60] Cross NE, Glantz ME. Neurologic complications of radiation therapy. Neurol Clin 2003;21:249–77.

[61] Beredjiklian PK, Drummond DS, Dormans JP, et al. Orthopedic manifestations of chronic graft-versus-host disease. J Pediatr Orthop 1998;18:572–5.

[62] Stevens AM, Sullivan KM, Nelson JL. Polymyositis as a manifestation of chronic graft-versus-host disease. Rheumatology (Oxford) 2003;42:34–9.

[63] Krouwer HGJ, Wijdicks EFM. Neurologic complications of bone marrow transplantation. Neurol Clin 2003;21:319–52.

[64] Amato AA, Barohn RJ, Sahenk Z, et al. Polyneuropathy complicating bone marrow and solid organ transplantation. Neurology 1993;43:1513–8.

[65] Wen PY, Alyea EP, Simon D, et al. Guillain-Barré syndrome following allogenic bone marrow transplantation. Neurology 1997;49:1711–4.

ELSEVIER
SAUNDERS

Phys Med Rehabil Clin N Am
19 (2008) 47–59

PHYSICAL MEDICINE
AND REHABILITATION
CLINICS OF
NORTH AMERICA

Neuromuscular Complications of Statins

Sung C. Ahn, DO[a,b,]*

[a]*943 Hayes Avenue, Oak Park, IL 60302-1411, USA*
[b]*Loyola University, 2160 South 1st Avenue, Maywood, IL 60153-5500, USA*

Statins, 3-hydroxy-3-methlglutaryl coenzyme A (HMG-CoA) reductase inhibitors, are commonly prescribed for patients who have hyperlipidemia. Statins were first approved for use in 1987. Statin therapy is well documented to reduce serum low-density lipoprotein (LDL) levels, incidence of cardiovascular events, and mortality [1–3]. Although statin therapy is well tolerated, serious adverse affects have been reported, including neuromuscular and hepatic complications. Myopathy is particularly concerning because of the potential for rhabdomyolysis and death. Recently peripheral neuropathy also has been identified as a possible complication. The incidence of neuromuscular complications is expected to increase with the increased number of people using statin therapy. Clinicians should be aware of the potential neuromuscular complications. This article reviews epidemiology, possible mechanisms, risk factors, and management of statin-associated neuromuscular complications.

Epidemiology of statin-induced myopathy

The exact incidence of statin-associated myopathy is difficult to assess because of the various definitions of myopathy used in describing this problem in the literature. Clinicians should be aware of the different terminology. "Myopathy" is defined as any muscle pain or problem. "Myalgia" refers to muscle aches and pains without elevation of serum creatine kinase (CK) levels. "Myositis" includes CK elevation with muscle discomfort. "Rhabdomyolysis" is muscle complaint with CK elevation greater than 10 times the normal upper limit (UNL) [4].

Given these limitations, the incidence of statin myopathy is approximately 1% to 5% of patients who are on statin therapy [4–6]. Overall the incidence of rhabdomyolysis is 1.6 to 6.5 per 100,000 persons per year for monotherapy,

---

* Loyola University, 2160 South 1st Avenue, Maywood, IL 60153-5500.
E-mail address: ahn.sungchul@mayo.edu

1047-9651/08/$ - see front matter © 2008 Elsevier Inc. All rights reserved.
doi:10.1016/j.pmr.2007.10.002
pmr.theclinics.com

with the exception of cerivastatin [7]. The incidence for cerivastatin is 10 times greater than other statin monotherapy [5]. The incidence of rhabdomyolysis increases to 5.98 per 10,000 persons per year when the statin is combined with fibrate [5]. Combination of statin with gemfibrozil has a 15 times higher incidence of rhabdomyolysis than with fenofibrate [8].

Fatality from rhabdomyolysis is 10% [7]. The death rate for statin-associated myopathy has been reported as 0.15 per 1 million prescriptions [9]. Cerivastatin is reported to have 16 to 80 times higher incidence of fatal rhabdomyolysis than other statins and was withdrawn from the market in August 2001 [10]. Discussion of cerivastatin is limited here because it is no longer available.

Currently there are several types of statins on the market: fluvastatin (Lescol), pravastatin (Pravachol), atorvastatin (Lipitor), simvastatin (Zocor), lovastatin (Mevacor), and rosuvastatin (Crestor). All the statins except fluvastatin have reports of fatal cases of rhabdomyolysis ranging from 3 to 19 cases [10]. The incidence of rhabdomyolysis for lovastatin, atorvastatin, and simvastatin is approximately 4 per 100,000 person-years, whereas for pravastatin it is 1 per 100,000 per year [7]. Statistically there is no difference in the incidence of rhabdomyolysis between these statins. Fatal rhabdomyolysis has not been reported when fluvastatin is used alone. A recent case report, however, showed that a combination of fluvastatin and gemfibrozil can lead to rhabdomyolysis [11]. Use of either fluvastatin or pravastatin seems to have a safety advantage, but they are less effective in lowering serum LDL levels [7].

Mechanism of statin-induced myopathy

The precise mechanism of statin-induced myopathy is unclear. One theory is that statins may have cholesterol-independent or pleiotropic effects. Statins reversibly inhibit HMG-CoA reductase, which is the rate-limiting enzyme for cholesterol synthesis. HMG-CoA reductase converts HMG-CoA to mevalonate. Mevalonate is an essential component in cholesterol synthesis. Mevalonate is also an intermediate for many other metabolites, including isoprenylated pyrophosphate (IPP). This leads to formation of farnesylated pyrophosphate and geranylgeranyl pyrophosphate [12–14]. Farnesyl pyrophosphate leads to formation of farnesylated protein (Ras) and ubiquinone (coenzyme Q10). Geranylgeranyl pyrophosphate leads to the formation of geranylgeranylated proteins (Rho) [15]. The Ras and Rho play an important role in cellular differentiation, proliferation, and cell stability [6,16,17]. Statins are hypothesized to reduce Ras and Rho. As a result, muscle cells may be impaired in cellular differentiation, proliferation, and cell stability, and this may lead to myopathy. The reduction of Ras and Rho also increases cytosolic calcium, which increases the activation of apoptosis by way of the mitochondrial transition pore [15]. Another theory is that statin therapy increases apoptosis in skeletal muscle, which may lead to the clinical presentation of myopathy [15].

In addition to these pleiotropic metabolic consequences, statins may also have effects on ubiquinones, such as coenzyme Q10 (Co Q10) [18]. Ubiquinone is an antioxidant and membrane stabilizer that is an essential cofactor in the electron transport chain in mitochondria, where adenosine triphosphate (ATP) is generated [10,18]. By reducing the production of ubiquinone, the energy source may get impaired, which may lead to impaired metabolism in myocytes [19]. This may lead to membrane instability and to myopathy. The evidence of this is marginal, however. One study showed no difference in ubiquinone concentration in patients receiving simvastatin (20 mg/day) for 6 months compared with the control group as demonstrated by muscle biopsy [20]. Another recent research study showed that statin may cause a mild reduction of CoQ10 in muscle, but not enough to cause myopathy [21]. In that study, CoQ10 level was measured from muscle biopsy of 18 patients who had proven statin-related myopathy. The results showed muscle CoQ10 concentration was not statistically different between the statin and control groups, although the absolute level was slightly lower in the statin group. Three patients had CoQ10 levels greater than 2 standard deviations below the lower limit of normal. Fourteen of 18 patients had normal muscle structure [21]. In contrast, another recent study involving 48 patients showed that muscle ubiquinone concentration was significantly lower in the simvastatin group than in the placebo group [22]. Given the mixed results of the studies to date, low ubiquinone is not clearly defined as a cause for statin-induced myopathy; however, some clinicians found that ubiquinone supplements have improved the myalgia symptoms that started after statin therapy [23,24]. Further research on ubiquinone is necessary to clarify the significance of ubiquinone supplementation and statin-associated myopathy.

Another theory is that hydrophilic statins may have a lower risk for myopathy than hydrophobic statins. Statins enter cells by high lipid solubility or by active transport. One of the important transport systems is the organic anion transporting polypeptide 1B1 (OATP), which actively takes up the statin into hepatocytes. The statins are most effective in the hepatocytes. Human muscles do not have OATP active transporters. Statins thus need to enter muscle cells by lipid solubility. If the statin is hydrophilic (less lipid soluble), the statin is therefore less likely to enter the muscle cell and less likely to cause myotoxicity [6]. Among the statins, pravastatin and rosuvastatin are the most hydrophilic statins [9].These statins, however, have been reported to cause myopathy [25]. The theory that hydrophilic statins have a protective effect against myopathy is plausible but has not been clearly proven, and further studies need to be done [9,26].

Risk factors for statin-induced myopathy

Several factors can increase risk for statin-associated myopathy. Patient characteristics that include advanced age (greater than 65 years), female gender, and small body habitus have been reported as risk factors [1,4,10].

Comorbid conditions, such as hypothyroidism, chronic renal disease, hepatic dysfunction, and diabetes, can also increase the risk for myopathy [27]. When the statin is given to hypothyroid patients, the patient's CK level can be increased and may cause myopathy [28].

The risk can also be increased with increased concentration of serum statin in the peripheral blood and muscle cells [4,29,30].The statin concentration, however, is not linearly correlated with the incidence of myotoxicity. One significant way to increase serum statin concentration is drug–drug interactions with the statin. Statin monotherapy rarely causes myopathy that leads to rhabdomyolysis, but concomitant medications metabolized by the cytochrome P450 (CYP) pathway seem to increase the risk for myopathy. Most statins are metabolized by CYP enzymes. Specifically, simvastatin, lovastatin, and atorvastatin are metabolized primarily by CYP 3A4 and some CYP 2C8 enzymes [30]. Fluvastatin and rosuvastatin are metabolized by CYP2C9 enzymes. Pravastatin is the only statin that is metabolized by a non-CYP enzyme [30]. Administration of medications that inhibit CYP 3A4 enzymes reduces the metabolism of simvastatin, lovastatin, and atorvastatin. As a result, these statin concentrations are increased. For example, itraconazole inhibits CYP 3A4 enzyme, and it is known to increase the concentration of simvastatin and lovastatin [6,30]. Studies also show that some CYP3A4 inhibitors are more potent than others. Ritonavir, itraconazole, and ketoconazole are considered strong CYP3A4 inhibitors [30]. Erythromycin, clarithromycin, telithromycin, verapamil, and diltiazem are considered potent CYP inhibitors. Table 1 outlines common medications that increase the risk for myopathy with concomitant use of statins. Many reports showed that the combination of simvastatin, lovastatin, or atorvastatin with CYP 3A4 inhibitor led to rhabdomyolysis [1,5,30].

Not only can medications inhibit the CYP3A4, but grapefruit juice can inhibit CYP3A4 enzymes. Recent studies show that regular grapefruit juice intake can increase the atorvastatin, lovastatin, and simvastatin concentration from three- to fourfold up to as high as 10-fold [31–33]. Grapefruit juice does not seem to increase pravastatin concentration [30], most likely because pravastatin is not metabolized by way of the CYP pathway. One case report associated statin-associated rhabdomyolysis with daily grapefruit juice consumption [34]. The patient was asymptomatic while taking simvastatin, but developed myopathic symptoms with serum CK of 12,640 U/L after daily grapefruit juice consumption [34]. Because grapefruit juice intake has long been considered a technique to reduce cholesterol, the interaction with statin therapy is important to remember.

Another way that serum statin concentration is increased is through inhibition of its metabolism. The glucuronidation pathway is necessary for statin metabolism. Statin elimination is reduced with inhibition of the glucuronidation pathway. Gemfibrozil is reported to inhibit the glucuronidation pathway, and this may slow statin elimination, thereby increasing the statin serum concentration [35,36]. Increased serum statin concentration

Table 1
Inhibitors of the cytochrome P450 enzymatic pathway

	CYP3A4	CYP2C9
CYP substrates (statins)	Atorvastatin	Fluvastatin
	Lovastatin	Rosuvastatin (2C19-minor)
	Simvastatin	
Inhibitors	Ketoconazole	Ketoconazole
	Itraconazole	Fluconazole
	Fluconazole	Sulfaphenazole
	Erythromycin	
	Clarithromycin	
	Tricyclic antidepressants	
	Nefazodone	
	Venlafaxine	
	Fluvoxamine	
	Fluoxetine	
	Sertraline	
	Cyclosporine A	
	Tacrolimus	
	Mibefradil	
	Diltiazem	
	Verapamil	
	Protease inhibitors	
	Midazolam	
	Corticosteroids	
	Grapefruit juice	
	Tamoxifen	
	Amiodarone	

(*Data from* Bellosta S, Paoletti R, et al. Safety of statins focus on clinical pharmacokinetics and drug interactions. Circulation 2004;109(Suppl III):50–7.)

increases the risk for myopathy. The combination of gemfibrozil and statin is known to increase myotoxicity [30]. Jones and Davidson [8] reported that the combination of gemfibrozil with statins other than cerivastatin caused rhabdomyolysis in 8.6 per 1 million prescriptions. The combination of fenofibrate and statins associated with rhabdomyolysis in only 0.58 per 1 million prescriptions. One main reason for this difference is that fenofibrate does not significantly inhibit the glucuronidation pathway, whereas gemfibrozil does [36]. As a result, statin serum concentration may be high in the gemfibrozil group, and this can lead to myopathy.

Clinical presentation of statin-associated myopathy

Patients who have statin-associated myopathy present with a wide clinical spectrum, from minimal muscle pain to frank rhabdomyolysis. One study reports that most patients complain of diffuse muscle pain with weakness (1 out of three patients) [37]. This study found that the duration of statin therapy before onset of myopathy symptoms was 6.3 months, and the symptoms lasted 2.3 months after the statin was discontinued.

Approximately 65% of patients had elevated serum CK level, with a mean value of 10,160 U/L, median value of 328 U/L, a wide range from as low as 36 up to140,190 U/L [37].Recent reports indicate that statin may cause myopathy with normal serum CK levels [38,39]. Phillips and colleagues [38] reported that patients who were on statin therapy had reduced strength consistent with myopathy. In addition, the muscle biopsy showed mitochondrial dysfunction consistent with myopathy. These patients, however, had normal serum CK levels. When the statin therapy was discontinued, the patient's strength returned, and the repeated muscle biopsy was normalized [38].

Electromyography (EMG) may have a role in assessing statin-associated myopathy. Most of these patients improve with cessation of statin therapy. In addition, the needle EMG findings may be normal, because the statin-associated myopathy predominantly affects type II muscle fibers [40,41]. Another study, however, showed needle EMG findings are not always normal in this population [21]. In one study, 40%, 40%, and 20% of patients had normal, myopathic, and neurogenic needle EMG findings, respectively [21]. The usefulness of the needle EMG is unclear in statin-associated myopathy because of the various needle EMG findings. The needle EMG may be helpful, however, if the symptoms do not improve or if another diagnosis is considered [41]. EMG can help determine if other causes of myopathy are present and should certainly be considered in the presence of clinical weakness or if cessation of statin therapy does not improve symptoms.

Muscle biopsy has little role in statin-associated myopathy. Most of these patients do not require muscle biopsy, because myopathic symptoms improve after discontinuation of statin therapy. The resolution takes approximately 2 months. One study showed that three patients who had statin-associated myopathy underwent muscle biopsy [38]. The biopsy showed intramuscular lipid accumulation consistent with mitochondrial myopathy [38]. After discontinuation of the statin therapy, the repeated muscle biopsy was normal or approaching normal [38]. Another study evaluated 48 patients who had hypercholesterolemia who were divided into three groups: simvastatin (80 mg/day), atorvastatin (40 mg/day), and placebo groups [22]. These patients had a quadriceps femoris muscle biopsy done before and after 8 weeks of treatment. The results showed that the patients in the simvastatin group had a 38% increased cholesterol concentration in the muscle cells, whereas the atorvastatin and placebo groups did not have any change [22]. None of these patients developed myopathic symptoms. This study suggests that not all the statins have the same impact on the cholesterol concentration in the muscle cell. Muscle biopsy does not show distinctive characteristics specific for statin-induced myopathy. Further study is needed to demonstrate muscle biopsy usefulness in these patients. Like needle EMG, muscle biopsy may be useful if the myopathic symptoms continue despite stopping the statin therapy or in cases in which another diagnosis is considered.

Management of statin-associated myopathy

Prevention is the first line of management in patients who have statin-associated myopathy. One obvious method of prevention is to avoid using statin therapy. One can lower the LDL level by diet and exercise. Another way to reduce the risk for myopathy is to use the minimum statin dose needed to achieve a therapeutic LDL level [4]. The statin dose may need to be adjusted based on the risk–benefit ratio for each patient. For example, advanced age, female gender, small body habitus, chronic renal disease, diabetes, and concomitant CYP-metabolized medications are documented to increase the risk for myopathy [4]. Currently there is no specific dose adjustment for each risk factor, but clinicians need to be cautious and start at the lowest dose. In addition to considering the risk factors, clinicians may choose to use the most effective statin to minimize the statin dose. Not all the statins have the same efficacy. A recent study compared the efficacy of rosuvastatin, atorvastatin, simvastatin, and pravastatin for reducing serum LDL and increasing HDL levels [42]. The study included 2431 adults who had hypercholesterolemia and who were randomly assigned to each group. The statin dose ranged from 10 to 80 mg, and the subjects took the statin for 6 weeks. The study found rosuvastatin more effective in reducing serum LDL and increasing HDL levels compared with atorvastatin, pravastatin, and simvastatin. As the statin dose increased, the efficacy of decreasing LDL and increasing HDL levels also increased. Increasing the statin dose, however, also increased the risk for myopathy. Clinicians may use statin efficacy to maximize the benefit while minimizing the risk for patients.

Because most of rhabdomyolysis and serious myopathy occur with combinations of statin and concomitant medications, clinicians need to review drug interactions carefully. See Table 1 for common medications that may increase the risk for statin-induced myopathy. For example, some clinicians may start gemfibrate in addition to statin therapy to treat severe dyslipidemia. Gemfibrate is known to cause myopathy by itself, however, and it significantly increases risk for myopathy if used in combination with statins [5].There is a much lower incidence of myopathy when statins are combined with fenobride as compared with its combination with gemfibrate [8,35]. A recent study found that the number of rhabdomyolysis cases for combination of statin other than cerivastatin with fenofibrate was 0.58 per 1 million prescriptions, whereas the combination with gemfibrozil was 8.6 per 1 million prescriptions [8]. This finding is most likely attributable to gemfibrate inhibiting the glucuronidation pathway, as discussed. Fenofibrate does not inhibit the glucuronidation pathway. Clinicians can use this information to choose fenofibrate rather than gemfibrate to treat dyslipidemia in patients who are already on statin therapy.

Another common drug that interacts with statins is cyclosporine. Cyclosporine is often used in patients who receive transplants for immunosuppression. It is metabolized by CYP4A3 pathway, as is simvastatin, lovastatin, and atorvastatin. When cyclosporine is combined with one of these statins, the serum statin concentration may be increased, which leads to increased risk for myopathy. In some cases, patients cannot avoid combination therapy and may need to be monitored frequently for adverse affects, or clinicians can choose a statin that is metabolized by a non-CYP pathway, such as pravastatin. Patients should be aware of the greater risk for myopathy with the increased dose of statin and concomitant therapy that may interfere with statin metabolism. By knowing the risk factors, clinicians may follow patients even more closely for any adverse affects. Serious adverse outcomes can therefore be prevented.

Another way to reduce serious adverse effects is to educate patients about the symptoms of myopathy, such as myalgia, weakness, fatigue, cramps, and hemoglobinuria, before the statin is initiated. This may prompt the patient to seek medical attention, which leads to the proper diagnostic work-up. This may possibly reduce or prevent more serious adverse affects, such as rhabdomyolysis and death.

Conducting baseline lipid profile, CK, and liver function studies (including alanine transferase and aspartate transferase) is recommended before initiating statin therapy [4]. Based on these results, clinicians may decide whether to start the statin therapy or not. For instance, if the patient has a significantly elevated serum CK level, clinicians need to reassess the risks and benefits of statin therapy in addition to investigating the elevated CK level. The baseline laboratory results are also helpful when patients develop symptoms and signs of statin adverse affects. If patients develop myopathic symptoms, then clinicians can repeat the serum CK level to compare with the baseline CK level. This helps determine if the statin therapy has contributed to the abnormal results. Routine laboratory tests on asymptomatic patients, however, have little value [43]. One study found that only 2 of 1194 patients who were taking statin showed moderately elevated CK level (2.5–5.0 times normal) 1 [43]. The serum CK level is a marker for muscle damage, but patients who have statin-associated myopathy may have normal serum CK levels, as noted [38,39].

If a patient develops myopathic signs and symptoms, a repeat CK level and a thyroid-stimulating hormone level are recommended [4]. Clinicians should exclude any physical activity etiology, because moderate physical activity can increase serum CK levels [4]. For example, Thompson and colleagues [44] showed that subjects who were taking lovastatin for 5 weeks had 62% and 77% higher CK levels at 24 and 48 hours after 45 minutes of treadmill exercise, respectively. If the CK level is greater than 10 times the upper limit of normal and the patient is symptomatic, statin therapy must be discontinued (Fig. 1). If the CK level is normal or moderately elevated (3–10 times UNL) and the patient is symptomatic, clinicians may choose to monitor the symptoms and CK level weekly. If the serial CK levels continue to increase with myopathic symptoms, clinicians should discontinue the statin therapy or reduce the statin dose [4]. Although routine CK levels

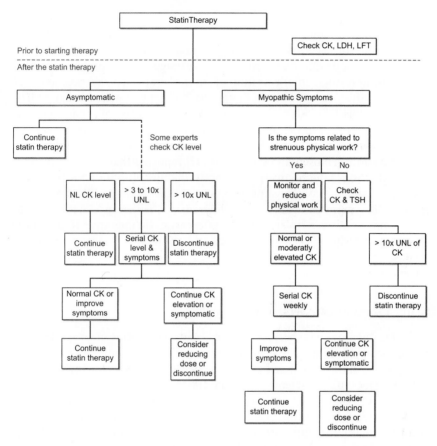

Fig. 1. Statin therapy. NL, normal; CK, creatine kinase; TSH, thyroid stimulating hormone; UNL, upper normal limit; LDH, low density lipoprotein; LFT, liver function test.

in asymptomatic patients do not have clear usefulness, some clinicians do check CK levels. If the CK level is greater than 10 times the UNL in asymptomatic patients, the statin therapy should be discontinued [4]. If the CK level is moderately elevated (3–10 times UNL), consider serial CK levels. If these patients become symptomatic and the CK level continues to increase, discontinue the statin therapy or decrease the statin dose.

Some experts believe the CoQ10 supplement has a role in preventing or alleviating myopathic symptoms and therefore in treating patients who have statin-induced myopathy with CoQ10 [24]. One study evaluated 50 patients who stopped statin therapy because of adverse affects, such as myalgia, fatigue, dyspnea, memory loss, and peripheral neuropathy [24]. These patients were treated with a CoQ10 supplement with resulting improvement in all of these categories.I It was not clear, however, whether the symptoms improved because the statin therapy was stopped or because CoQ10 supplement was initiated. Future research is recommended to evaluate if combined statin therapy and CoQ10 supplementation reduces the number of myopathic complaints compared to those patients on statin therapy alone.

Treatment of patients who have statin-associated myopathy includes stopping the medication with supportive management. Most patients fully recover from myalgia after cessation of statin therapy. The average duration of myalgia after stopping statin therapy is 2.3 months, with a range of 0.25 to 14.0 months [37]. After the resolution of the myopathic symptoms, re-challenging with statin therapy is a possibility. There is no specific guideline for rechallenging with statin therapy. The patient may restart a different or the same statin. Hansen and colleagues [37] reported that 37 of 45 patients who had statin-induced myopathy received different statin therapy after resolution of myopathic symptoms. Of these 37 patients, 21 experienced myopathic symptoms again with a different statin therapy. Sixteen of the 37 patients, however, tolerated the different statin therapy. If the statin therapy has greater benefits than risks, rechallenging with statin therapy is a consideration. Clinicians, however, need to carefully monitor for further adverse affects.

Statin-associated peripheral neuropathy

Statin therapy has been associated with peripheral neuropathy, but limited studies are available at this time. A recent report states that the incidence of statin-associated peripheral neuropathy is 1 per 14,000 people per year [45], and prevalence is 60 per 100,000 [7]. The risk for peripheral neuropathy is high if patients are on statin therapy for greater than 2 years [46,47]. A Danish case-control study reports that the relative risk for peripheral neuropathy for statin users is 2.5 times higher than in the general population [47]. Another article, however, pointed out that this study has flaws and questions the validity of the conclusion [48]. Because statin-induced peripheral neuropathy is rare and general peripheral neuropathy is associated with many risk factors, a precise incidence and prevalence of statin-induced peripheral neuropathy is challenging. In general, statin therapy's benefit far outweighs the risk for peripheral neuropathy.

The mechanism of statin-induced peripheral neuropathy is unknown. Statins interfere with cholesterol synthesis by inhibiting HMG-CoA reductase. One theory is that interfering with cholesterol synthesis may alter the peripheral nerve membrane and its function [47]. As a result, these patients show clinical signs and symptoms of peripheral neuropathy. Not only do the statins interfere with cholesterol synthesis, but ubiquinone (CoQ10) synthesis may also be affected as discussed. The reduction of CoQ10, a mitochondrial respiratory chain enzyme, may reduce energy production for the neurons, which may lead to peripheral neuropathy [47]. These ideas remain theories only, and no confirming research studies have been done.

The presentation of statin-induced peripheral neuropathy is generally similar to that seen in patients who have non–statin-associated peripheral neuropathy. One study showed that most patients present with pain, numbness, and paresthesia [47]. This study suggested that motor fibers are more affected than sensory fibers, with mostly axonal involvement [47]. This suggestion, however, is based on only nine patients. Further study is needed to characterize statin-induced peripheral neuropathy.

Managing patients who have suspected statin-associated peripheral neuropathy is similar to managing patients who have statin-induced myopathy. Clinicians should confirm the diagnosis of peripheral neuropathy by history, physical examination, and possibly diagnostic tests, such as electrophysiologic studies. Other more common causes of peripheral neuropathy must be excluded, although, because the etiology of many peripheral neuropathies remains elusive, this is challenging. After excluding other etiologies, one should consider discontinuing statin therapy to see if neurologic symptoms resolve. Most of the peripheral neuropathy symptoms resolve from immediately to over 15 to 18 months, after cessation of statin therapy [45]. At that time, one could restart with alternative statin therapy or rechallenge. Because there are a limited number of cases available, a specific recommendation cannot be made. Again, the risk factors associated with elevated lipids must be weighed against the potential risks associated with statin therapy.

Summary

Statin therapy is widely accepted to reduce cardiovascular events and mortality. Fortunately statin therapy is well tolerated, but clinicians should be aware of the risk for myopathy, rhabdomyolysis, and, rarely, peripheral neuropathy as complications. As more people use statin therapy, the incidence of these adverse affects will likely increase. Clinicians may be able to detect the neuromuscular complications early and prevent more severe complications. Further research is necessary to better understand the etiology and management of statin-related neuromuscular disease.

References

[1] Ballantyne CM, Corsini A, Davidson MH, et al. Risk for myopathy with statin therapy in high-risk patients. Arch Intern Med 2003;163:553.

[2] Lewis SJ, Moye LA, Sacks FM, et al. Effect of pravastatin on cardiovascular events in older patients with myocardial infarction and cholesterol levels in the average range. Results of the Cholesterol and Recurrent Events (CARE) trial. Ann Intern Med 1998;129:681.

[3] Sacks FM. High-intensity statin treatment for coronary heart disease. JAMA 2004;291:1132.

[4] Pasternak R. ACC/AHA/NHLBI clinical advisory on the use and safety of statins [see comment]. Stroke 2002;33:2337.

[5] Graham DJ, Staffa JA, Shatin D, et al. Incidence of hospitalized rhabdomyolysis in patients treated with lipid-lowering drugs [see comment]. JAMA 2004;292:2585.

[6] Thompson PD, Clarkson P, Karas RH. Statin-associated myopathy. JAMA 2003;289:1681.

[7] Law M, Rudnicka AR. Statin safety: a systematic review. Am J Cardiol 2006;97:52C.

[8] Jones PH, Davidson MH. Reporting rate of rhabdomyolysis with fenofibrate + statin versus gemfibrozil + any statin. Am J Cardiol 2005;95:120.

[9] Bellosta S, Paoletti R, Corsini A. Safety of statins: focus on clinical pharmacokinetics and drug interactions. Circulation 2004;109:III50.

[10] Rosenson RS. Current overview of statin-induced myopathy. Am J Med 2004;116:408.

[11] Akoglu H, Yilmaz R, Kirkpantur A, et al. Combined organ failure with combination antihyperlipidemic treatment: a case of hepatic injury and acute renal failure. Ann Pharmacother 2007;41:143.

[12] Goldstein JL, Brown MS. Regulation of the mevalonate pathway. Nature 1990;343:425.

[13] Holstein SA, Wohlford-Lenane CL, Hohl RJ. Consequences of mevalonate depletion. Differential transcriptional, translational, and post-translational up-regulation of Ras, Rap1a, RhoA, and RhoB. J Biol Chem 2002;277:10678.

[14] Leonard S, Beck L, Sinensky M. Inhibition of isoprenoid biosynthesis and the post-translational modification of pro-p21. J Biol Chem 1990;265:5157.

[15] Dirks AJ, Jones KM. Statin-induced apoptosis and skeletal myopathy. Am J Physiol Cell Physiol 2006;291:C1208.

[16] Macaluso M, Russo G, Cinti C, et al. Ras family genes: an interesting link between cell cycle and cancer. J Cell Physiol 2002;192:125.

[17] Olsson AG. Expanding options with a wider range of rosuvastatin doses. Clin Ther 2006;28:1747.

[18] Baker SK, Tarnopolsky MA. Statin myopathies: pathophysiologic and clinical perspectives. Clin Invest Med 2001;24:258.

[19] Bliznakov EG. Lipid-lowering drugs (statins), cholesterol, and coenzyme Q10. The Baycol case a modern Pandora's box. Biomed Pharmacother 2002;56:56.

[20] Laaksonen R, Jokelainen K, Laakso J, et al. The effect of simvastatin treatment on natural antioxidants in low-density lipoproteins and high-energy phosphates and ubiquinone in skeletal muscle. Am J Cardiol 1996;77:851.

[21] Lamperti C, Naini AB, Lucchini V, et al. Muscle coenzyme Q10 level in statin-related myopathy. Arch Neurol 2005;62:1709.

[22] Paiva H, Thelen KM, Van Coster R, et al. High-dose statins and skeletal muscle metabolism in humans: a randomized, controlled trial. Clin Pharmacol Ther 2005;78:60.

[23] Koumis T, Nathan JP, Rosenberg JM, et al. Strategies for the prevention and treatment of statin-induced myopathy: is there a role for ubiquinone supplementation? Am J Health Syst Pharm 2004;61:515.

[24] Langsjoen PH, Langsjoen JO, Langsjoen AM, et al. Treatment of statin adverse effects with supplemental coenzyme Q10 and statin drug discontinuation. Biofactors 2005;25:147.

[25] Thompson PD, Clarkson PM, Rosenson RS, et al. An assessment of statin safety by muscle experts. Am J Cardiol 2006;97:17.

[26] Alsheikh-Ali AA, Karas RH. Safety of lovastatin/extended release niacin compared with lovastatin alone, atorvastatin alone, pravastatin alone, and simvastatin alone (from the United States Food and Drug Administration Adverse Event Reporting System). Am J Cardiol 2007;99:379.

[27] Talbert RL. Safety issues with statin therapy. J Am Pharm Assoc 2006;46:479.

[28] Tokinaga K, Oeda T, Suzuki Y, et al. HMG-CoA reductase inhibitors (statins) might cause high elevations of creatine phosphokinase (CK) in patients with unnoticed hypothyroidism. Endocr J 2006;53:401.

[29] Evans M, Rees A. The myotoxicity of statins. Curr Opin Lipidol 2002;13:415.

[30] Neuvonen PJ, Niemi M, Backman JT. Drug interactions with lipid-lowering drugs: mechanisms and clinical relevance. Clin Pharmacol Ther 2006;80:565.

[31] Ando H, Tsuruoka S, Yanagihara H, et al. Effects of grapefruit juice on the pharmacokinetics of pitavastatin and atorvastatin. Br J Clin Pharmacol 2005;60:494.

[32] Kantola T, Kivisto KT, Neuvonen PJ. Grapefruit juice greatly increases serum concentrations of lovastatin and lovastatin acid [see comment]. Clin Pharmacol Ther 1998;63:397.

[33] Lilja JJ, Neuvonen M, Neuvonen PJ. Effects of regular consumption of grapefruit juice on the pharmacokinetics of simvastatin. Br J Clin Pharmacol 2004;58:56.

[34] Dreier JP, Endres M. Statin-associated rhabdomyolysis triggered by grapefruit consumption. Neurology 2004;62:670.

[35] Owczarek J, Jasinska M, Orszulak-Michalak D. Drug-induced myopathies. An overview of the possible mechanisms. Pharmacol Rep 2005;57:23.

[36] Prueksaritanont T, Tang C, Qiu Y, et al. Effects of fibrates on metabolism of statins in human hepatocytes. Drug Metab Dispos 2002;30:1280.

[37] Hansen KE, Hildebrand JP, Ferguson EE, et al. Outcomes in 45 patients with statin-associated myopathy [see comment]. Arch Intern Med 2005;165:2671.

[38] Phillips PS, Haas RH, Bannykh S, et al. Statin-associated myopathy with normal creatine kinase levels [see comment]. Ann Intern Med 2002;137:581.

[39] Troseid M, Henriksen OA, Lindal S. Statin-associated myopathy with normal creatine kinase levels. Case report from a Norwegian family. Apmis 2005;113:635.

[40] Sinzinger H, Wolfram R, Peskar BA. Muscular side effects of statins. J Cardiovasc Pharmacol 2002;40:163.

[41] Strommen JA, Johns JS, Kim CT, et al. Neuromuscular rehabilitation and electrodiagnosis. 3. Diseases of muscles and neuromuscular junction. Arch Phys Med Rehabil 2005;86:S18.

[42] Jones PH, Davidson MH, Stein EA, et al. Comparison of the efficacy and safety of rosuvastatin versus atorvastatin, simvastatin, and pravastatin across doses (STELLAR* Trial). Am J Cardiol 2003;92:152.

[43] Smith CC, Bernstein LI, Davis RB, et al. Screening for statin-related toxicity: the yield of transaminase and creatine kinase measurements in a primary care setting [see comment]. Arch Intern Med 2003;163:688.

[44] Thompson PD, Zmuda JM, Domalik LJ, et al. Lovastatin increases exercise-induced skeletal muscle injury. Metabolism 1997;46:1206.

[45] Chong PH, Boskovich A, Stevkovic N, et al. Statin-associated peripheral neuropathy: review of the literature. Pharmacotherapy 2004;24:1194.

[46] de Langen JJ, van Puijenbroek EP. HMG-CoA-reductase inhibitors and neuropathy: reports to the Netherlands Pharmacovigilance Centre. N J Med 2006;64:334.

[47] Gaist D, Jeppesen U, Andersen M, et al. Statins and risk of polyneuropathy: a case-control study [see comment]. Neurology 2002;58:1333.

[48] Leis AA, Stokic DS, Olivier J. Statins and polyneuropathy: setting the record straight. Muscle Nerve 2005;32:428.

ELSEVIER
SAUNDERS

Phys Med Rehabil Clin N Am
19 (2008) 61–79

PHYSICAL MEDICINE
AND REHABILITATION
CLINICS OF
NORTH AMERICA

Neuromuscular Disorders Associated with Paraproteinemia

Charlene Hoffman-Snyder, CNP*,
Benn E. Smith, MD

*Department of Neurology, Mayo Clinic,
13400 East Shea Boulevard, Scottsdale, AZ 85259, USA*

The broad spectrum of plasma cell dyscrasias characterized as paraproteinemias or monoclonal gammopathies is subclassified by proliferation of particular individual clones of β lymphocytes that secrete excess monoclonal antibodies. This overproduction of plasma cells can be either neoplastic or a low-grade potentially neoplastic process. Monoclonal proteins are prevalent in 3% of the general population older than 50 years of age, with rates increasing with age. Prevalence rates are higher for men than women, and African Americans have a threefold higher age-adjusted prevalence rate than Caucasian persons [1,2].

Paraproteinemias are usually asymptomatic and are found on routine blood testing without associated abnormalities. Nevertheless, certain disease associations occur more often than by chance and include: (1) monoclonal gammopathies of undetermined significance (MGUS), biclonal gammopathies, idiopathic Bence Jones proteinuria; (2) the malignant monoclonal gammopathies of multiple myeloma, smoldering multiple myeloma, Waldenström macroglobulinemia, uncommon malignant disorders of solitary plasmacytoma, and POEMS syndrome (*p*olyneuropathy, *o*rganomegaly, *e*ndocrinopathy, *m*onoclonal gammopathy, and *s*kin changes); (3) systemic AL (immunoglobulin light chain) amyloidosis; (4) cryoglobulinemia; and (5) heavy-chain diseases [3]. When clinical features are present, they range from fatigue, weight loss, purpura, congestive heart failure, nephrotic syndrome, peripheral neuropathy, and orthostatic hypotension, to mucocutaneous bleeding [3].

---

* Corresponding author.
E-mail address: snyder.charlene@mayo.edu (C. Hoffman-Snyder).

1047-9651/08/$ - see front matter © 2008 Elsevier Inc. All rights reserved.
doi:10.1016/j.pmr.2007.10.005   *pmr.theclinics.com*

Paraprotein-associated neuropathies have emerged as an important category of late-onset chronic polyneuropathies, warranting further evaluation for an underlying plasma cell dyscrasia [4]. In patients presenting with peripheral neuropathy of unknown cause, 10% will have a monoclonal protein, the majority of whom will be found to have MGUS. This is of even greater importance in patients with patterns of nerve conduction abnormality suggestive of demyelination, autonomic dysfunction, predominantly motor neuropathy, or lower motor neuron findings. The plasma cells disorders most often associated with neuropathy include MGUS, smoldering myeloma, multiple myeloma, Waldenström macroglobulinemia, solitary plasmacytoma, systemic AL amyloidosis and POEMS and are discussed later in this monograph [5].

It is helpful to distinguish between a monoclonal and a polyclonal process in plasma cell disorders, because unlike the monoclonal process, a reactive or inflammatory process commonly causes the polyclonal increase in immunoglobulin (Ig) [6]. Polyclonal immunoglobulins are created by many clones of plasma cells. Blood levels of polyclonal gamma globulin of 3 g/dL or more are associated with liver disease, connective tissue diseases, chronic infections, and nonhematologic malignancies [7].

The monoclonal process, however, is more often associated with premalignant or malignant disease than its polyclonal counterpart. There can be an overlap in antibody-mediated pathogenic mechanisms among these different monoclonal and polyclonal antibodies [8].

Monoclonal proteins (also called M proteins, myeloma proteins, or paraproteins) consist of two heavy polypeptide chains of the same class and subclass and two light polypeptide chains of the same type. The different monoclonal proteins are known by letters that correspond to the class of their heavy chains, which are designated by Greek alphabet characters: γ (gamma) in IgG, α (alpha) in IgA, μ (mu) in IgM, δ (delta) in immunoglobulin D (IgD), and ϵ (epsilon) in immunoglobulin E (IgE). There are four subclasses for IgG, two subclasses for IgA, and no subclasses for IgM, IgD, or IgE. The light-chain types are kappa (κ) and lambda (λ). Each of these monoclonal proteins is produced by a proliferation of single clonal population of plasma cells in the bone marrow. The mechanism of monoclonal expansion of a single Ig-secreting plasma cell population is unknown in most instances [4]. A review of the data by Kyle and Rajkumar [9], however, suggests in at least 50% of MGUS there is evidence of genomic instability on molecular genetic testing, including primary chromosomal translocations at the immunoglobulin heavy chain locus 14q32 (50%), hyperdiploidy (40%), or unknown (10%) [8,10–12]. The cause for this genomic instability is uncertain. Current evidence, however, suggests that antigenic stimulation related to infection and immune dysregulation may be an important factor [9]. Additional contributors to the progression of MGUS to multiple myeloma are under study and include changes in the microenvironment by way of induction of angiogenesis, suppression of cell-mediated immunity, adhesions of myeloma cells to stroma, alteration of adhesion molecules, and stromal cytokine overexpression [9].

Increased osteoclast activation and receptor activator of nuclear factor-kappa beta B ligand (RANKL) and decreased levels of osteoprotegerin (OPG) result in lytic bone lesions and osteoporosis [7,9,12]. The pathogenic link between the monoclonal proteins and nerve damage is known only in a few instances. In the IgM class it is believed that neuropathy is related to the reactivity of the circulating antibodies that are directed against specific neural antigens expressed on the peripheral nerves, such as myelin-associated glycoprotein (MAG), chondroitin sulfate, and sulfatide with consequential complement-dependent nerve damage [8]. Findings have shown that the deposition of IgM protein within the myelin in large and small myelinated fibers may have a role in the pathogenesis of neuropathy, although this remains unproven [5,13,14].

Recognition of monoclonal proteins

Identification of M proteins is best achieved by serum protein electrophoresis techniques. The immunofixation process distinguishes the immunoglobulin class and type of light chain. Densitometry is used to measure the monoclonal protein that is visible on serum electrophoresis and has replaced the use of nephelometry as a more reliable way to measure immunoglobulin levels. A 24-hour analysis of urine for protein excretion and a urine protein electrophoresis and immunofixation is warranted to detect and quantify the monoclonal protein in the urine. To date this has been the standard recommendation [15]. A recent study by Katzmann and colleagues [16] suggests this may not be necessary because of the highly sensitive serum free light-chain assay now available. Measurement of β_2-microglobulin has not proved predictive of malignant transformation and is no longer recommended. If a monoclonal protein is found, additional hematologic studies (serum calcium, complete blood count, and serum creatinine) are needed. Although a skeletal survey and aspirated bone marrow biopsy are generally performed to rule out myeloma, they are not considered necessary when other laboratory tests are normal and the serum monoclonal spike is less than 1.5 g per deciliter and other laboratory tests are normal [15]. If abnormalities are detected on these tests, appropriate tissue biopsy is recommended to exclude amyloidosis. When no monoclonal protein is uncovered, patients who have motor polyradiculoneuropathy with demyelinating features on nerve conduction studies should have cerebrospinal fluid examination, skeletal bone survey, and sural nerve biopsy (Fig. 1). Sural nerve biopsy has shown mixed pathology (fiber loss, segmental demyelination, and axonal degeneration). In the IgM class a predominantly demyelinating process is often observed. Patients who have progressive axonal neuropathies with autonomic dysfunction require biopsy of one or more appropriate tissues to rule out or confirm amyloidosis [17].

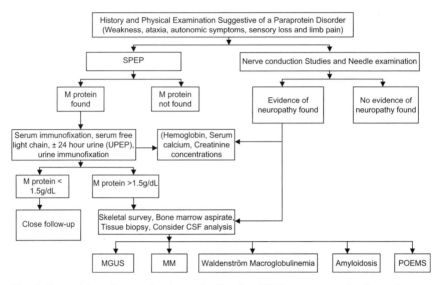

Fig. 1. Recognition of monoclonal protein disorder. SPEP, serum protein electrophoresis; CSF, cerebrospinal fluid; MGUS, monoclonal gammopathy of undetermined significance; MM, multiple myeloma; POEMS, polyneuropathy, organomegaly, endocrinopathy, monoclonal gammopathy and skin changes.

Electromyographic studies

Electromyographic changes in plasma cell disorders show abnormalities consistent with demyelination and axonal degeneration (Table 1). Nerve conductions are typically abnormal in motor and sensory fibers in the upper and lower extremities. Motor nerve conduction velocities are often decreased to less than the lower limits of normal by 20% or more. Sensory nerve action potentials are consistently reduced in amplitude or are unobtainable, with more pronounced changes in the lower limb nerves. Frequently F-wave latencies are prolonged but not out of proportion to the degree of peripheral nerve conduction slowing. In IgM neuropathies, the nerve conduction abnormalities tend to be more severe than the cases involving other protein classes. Needle examination demonstrates changes consistent with active denervation (increased insertional activity with fibrillation potentials) in more than 80% of patients. Evidence of coexisting demyelination and denervation is common. The sural sensory nerve more often shows damage than the median sensory nerve [4].

Monoclonal gammopathy of undetermined significance

MGUS is the most common plasma cell dyscrasia found in the general population and usually presents asymptomatically after the fifth decade of life [18]. It is considered a premalignant disorder characterized by limited monoclonal plasma cell proliferation in the bone marrow and absence of end-organ damage. In de novo paraproteinemia, approximately two thirds of the time after exclusion of amyloidosis, multiple or osteosclerotic myeloma, Waldenström macroglobulinemia, lymphoma, or lymphoproliferative disease, no identifiable cause is found, and the disorder by exclusion is classified as MGUS. Although characterized as premalignant, it is not truly benign in that it is linked to a lifelong risk for progression to multiple myeloma or related disorders, making lifelong follow-up necessary in all persons [19].

An M protein is found in 3% to 4% of patients who have a diffuse lymphoproliferative process, in the sera of patients who have chronic lymphocytic leukemia with no recognizable effect on the clinical course, in the dermatologic diseases of lichen myxedematosus, pyoderma gangrenosum, and necrobiotic xanthogranuloma, and more often in the peripheral neurologic disorders sensorimotor peripheral neuropathy and chronic inflammatory demyelinating polyneuropathy. MGUS occurs in approximately 5% to 10% of adult patients who have chronic idiopathic axonal polyneuropathy (CIAP), which represents a sixfold increase over the rate found in the general population [20].

The typical clinical presentations of the MGUS protein classes associated with chronic polyneuropathy are similar and usually begin in the sixth decade of life, progressing in a slow, insidious pattern as distal symmetric sensorimotor polyneuropathy. Sensory deficits begin in the toes and extend up the lower limbs to a greater extent than in the upper extremities. Muscle stretch reflexes are globally diminished or absent with almost universal sparing of cranial nerve function. Paresthesia, ataxia, and pain may be significant but seldom lead to complete inability to walk. The neuropathy in MGUS tends to be more relentlessly progressive than the typical relapsing–remitting course of chronic inflammatory demyelinating polyradiculoneuropathy (CIDP). Differentiating a patient who has MGUS from one who has another plasma cell disorder is difficult on clinical grounds alone. Use of laboratory and additional diagnostic study findings are often helpful in this regard. The recommended diagnostic criteria in patients who have suspected MGUS are summarized in Table 2. The initial studies to include are a compete blood count, serum creatinine, and serum calcium. If irregularities are identified in any of these tests, a plain film radiograph bone survey including long bones (the humerus and femur bilaterally) is done. A bone marrow aspirate and biopsy are recommended if the M-protein value is greater than or equal to 1.5 g/dL, if an IgA or an IgM MGUS is identified, or if a patient who has an abnormal serum free light chain (FLC) ratio is encountered [21].

Electrophysiologic studies often demonstrate findings suggesting demyelination or demyelination and axonal degeneration. In such cases motor nerve conduction velocities are reduced to less than the lower limits of normal, and sensory nerve action potentials are consistently reduced or unobtainable. Needle electromyography often shows changes consistent with denervation. Cerebrospinal fluid protein elevation can be seen, but there is no pleocytosis. Sural nerve biopsy studies of patients who have all

Table 1
Neuromuscular Axonal Disorders associated with Paraproteinemias

Disorder	Anatomical pattern	Nerve conduction changes	Pathological features	Paraprotein	Clinical features	Treatment
MGUS	DS, DSSP	Axonal	Axonal degeneration	IgM-κ or IgG-κ	Asymptomatic, neuropathy	Surveillance
Smoldering multiple myeloma	DS, DSSP	Axonal	Axonal degeneration, with or without amyloid deposition	IgM-κ or IgG-κ	Asymptomatic, neuropathy	Surveillance
Multiple myeloma	DS, DSSP	Axonal	Axonal degeneration, with or without amyloid deposition	IgM-κ or IgG-κ	Bone pain, fatigue, anemia, polyneuropathy, hypercalcemia, renal insufficiency	Irradiation, chemotherapy, autologous stem cell transplantation and novel drug trials (Thalidomide)
Solitary plasmacytoma	DS, DSSP	Axonal	Axonal degeneration, with or without amyloid deposition		Polyneuropathy, bone pain, solitary bone lesion	Resection and irradiation
POEMS syndrome	DS, DSSP areflexia simulates CIDP	Axonal, Demyelinating, similar to CIDP	Axonal, sclerotic bone lesions	IgG- λ or IgA-λ	Polyneuropathy, organomegaly, endocrinopathy, skin changes, peripheral edema, fatigue, papilledema, lymph node hyperplasia	Irradiation, autologous stem cell transplantation, melphalan plus prednisone
Waldenström macroglobulinemia	DS, DSSP a simulates CIDP	Axonal, demyelinating		IgM-κ	Fatigue, weight loss, oronasal bleeding, visual blurring, dyspnea, polyneuropathy, encephalopathy	Rituximab, nucleoside analogues, alkator agents

Systemic AL amyloidosis	S, A	Axonal	Axonal degeneration with amyloid deposition, rare myopathy	IgG-λ or IgA-λ	Chronic painful polyneuropathies, systemic organ involvement, rare proximal muscle weakness	Melphalan plus prednisone
MMN	S, SM	M	Lower motor neuron	IgM-GM1	Limb weakness, wasting predominantly in the arms	IVIg
Cryoglobulinemia	S, M, DSSP, SM, MM	Axonal	Axonal degeneration, vasculitis, inflammatory infiltrate	IgM or IgG	Arthralgias, purpura, leg ulcers, Raynaud's phenomenon, hepatosplenomegaly, painful polyneuropathies	For mild conservative measures. For severe plasma exchange, Prednisone, cytotoxic therapy

Abbreviations: MGUS, monoclonal gammopathy of undetermined significance; POEMS, polyneuropathy, organomegaly, endocrinopathy, IgM spike and skin changes; DSSP, distal symmetric sensorimotor polyneuropathies; MM, multiple mononeuropathies; SN, sensory neuronopathy or ganglionopathy; S, sensory neuropathy; M, motor neuropathy; A, autonomic neuropathy; CIDP, chronic inflammatory demyelinating polyneuropathy.

(*From* Ropper AH, Gorson KC. Neuropathies associated with paraproteinemia. N Engl J Med 1998;338(22):1602; with permission. Copyright © 1998, Massachusetts Medical Society.)

Table 2
Mayo Clinic diagnostic criteria for selected clonal plasma cell disorders

Disorder	Disease definition
MGUS	Serum monoclonal protein level <3 g/dL, bone marrow plasma cells <10%, and absence of end-organ damage, such as lytic bone lesions, anemia, hypercalcemia, or renal failure that can be attributed to a plasma cell proliferative disorder
SMM	Serum monoclonal protein (IgG or IgA) level ≥3 g/dL and bone marrow plasma cells >10%, absence of end, such as lytic bone lesions, anemia, hypercalcemia, or renal failure that can be attributed to a plasma cell proliferative disorder
Multiple myeloma	Bone marrow plasma cells ≥10%, presence of serum or urinary monoclonal protein (except in patients who have true nonsecretory multiple myeloma), plus evidence of lytic bone lesions, anemia, hypercalcemia, or renal failure that can be attributed to a plasma cell proliferative disorder
Waldenström macroglobulinemia	IgM monoclonal gammopathy (regardless of the size of the M protein) with >10% bone marrow lymphoplasmacytic infiltration (usually intertrabecular) by small lymphocytes that exhibit plasmacytoid or plasma cell differentiation a typical immunophenotype (eg, surface IgM⁺, CD5⁺/⁻, CD10⁻, CD19⁺, CD20⁺, CD23⁻, that satisfactorily excludes other lymphoproliferative disorders, including chronic leukemia and mantle cell lymphoma. Note: IgM MGUS is defined as serum IgM monoclonal protein level <3 g/dL, bone marrow lymphoplasmacytic infiltration <10%, and no evidence of anemia, constitutional symptoms, hyperviscosity, lymphadenopathy, or hepatosplenomegaly. Smoldering Waldenström macroglobulinemia (also referred to as indolent or asymptomatic Waldenström macroglobulinemia) is defined as serum IgM monoclonal protein level >3 g/dL and bone marrow lymphoplasmacytic infiltration >10% and no evidence of end-organ damage, such as anemia, constitutional symptoms, hyperviscosity, lymphadenopathy, or hepatosplenomegaly that can be attributed to a plasma cell proliferative disorder
Solitary plasmacytoma	Biopsy-proven solitary lesion of bone or soft tissue with evidence of clonal plasma cells, normal bone marrow with no evidence of clonal plasma cells, normal skeletal survey and MRI of spine and pelvis, absence of end-organ damage, such as lytic bone lesions, anemia, hypercalcemia, or renal failure that can be attributed to a plasma cell proliferative disorder
Systemic AL amyloidosis	Presence of an amyloid-related systemic syndrome (such as renal, liver, heart, gastrointestinal tract or peripheral nerve, or muscle involvement) with positive amyloid staining by Congo red or methyl violet in any tissue (eg, fat, aspiration bone marrow, or tissue biopsy), plus evidence that amyloid is light chain related established by direct examination of the amyloid (immunoperoxidase staining, direct sequencing, etc.) plus evidence of a monoclonal plasma cell proliferative disorder (serum and urine M protein, abnormal free light chain ratio, or clonal plasma cells in the bone marrow). Note: Approximately 2%–3% of patients who have AL amyloidosis will not meet the requirement for evidence of a monoclonal plasma cell disorder; the diagnosis of AL amyloidosis in these patients must be made with caution.

(Adapted from Rajkumar SV, Dispenzieri A, Kyle RA. Monoclonal gammopathy of undetermined significance, Waldenström macroglobulinemia, AL amyloidosis, and related plasma cell disorders: diagnosis and treatment. Mayo Clin Proc 2006;81(5):693–703; with permission.)

three monoclonal classes associated with neuropathy have shown mixed pathology [5].

The monoclonal proteins associated with MGUS and polyneuropathy belong to the IgM, IgG, and IgA heavy chain classes. The classes are often considered separately in research protocols and in clinical practice, because the clinical and laboratory features of IgG and IgA MGUS neuropathies may distinguish these conditions and their response to treatment [4]. IgM MGUS is distinguished from IgG and IgA by several features: it is over- represented in the neuropathy group when compared with the other classes, sensory ataxia occurs more frequently, and nerve conduction studies are more often demyelinating, significantly worse, and more frequently accompanied by dispersion of motor responses. Additionally, within the IgM MGUS group there is interest in the role that frequently associated antibodies (anti myelin-associated glycoprotein [MAG] antibody occurs in approximately 50% of patients who have IgM MGUS) may play in these neuropathies. The main idea is that should these antibodies prove to be pathogenic, treatments directed at antibody reduction may be efficacious. Additional monoclonal IgM antibodies react to other peripheral nerve antigens, including chondroitin sulfate C, sulfatide, cytoskeletal proteins, trisulfated heparin disaccharide, and various ganglioside moieties. These distinct characteristics raise the possibility of an antibody-mediated neuropathy. In the heavy chain class of IgG or IgA MGUS, clinical features can resemble CIDP, but because monoclonal proteins are not found in CIDP they are usually considered to be separate entities. Nonetheless, patients who have IgG and IgA MGUS have responded to plasma exchange, but those who have IgM MGUS have not [21].

Although MGUS is a common finding in clinical practice, determining whether it remains stable or progresses to multiple myeloma is a significant challenge. The rate of malignant progression is approximately 1% per year when other causes of death are factored in and is approximately 11% at 25 years. A risk stratification system (Table 3) can predict the risk for progression of MGUS based on three factors: size of the M-protein value being the most important predictor (the risk for progression of a serum M-protein of 1.5 g/L being twice the risk for progression with a value of 5 g/L); the type of immunoglobulin, and the serum FLC ratio [6,18,22]. Patients who have MGUS need indefinite monitoring with repeat serum protein electrophoresis (SPEP) every 6 to 12 months. Although the natural history of evolution of MGUS to malignancy is unknown, genetic changes, bone marrow angiogenesis, and various cytokines related to myeloma bone disease and possibly infectious agents may all play a part. The treatment for MGUS neuropathy is unclear. A decision to treat depends on the severity and temporal path of the neuropathy. An indolent course and minor deficits may mandate watchful waiting. If the neuropathy is severe and meets diagnostic criteria for CIDP, however, the patient may respond to immunomodulatory therapies. The response rates to plasmapheresis, intravenous immunoglobulins (IVIg), prednisone, or combinations have been promising. When there is a rapid

Table 3
Risk stratification model to predict progression of monoclonal gammopathy of undetermined
significance to myeloma or related disorders

Risk group	No. of patients	Relative risk 95% CL	Absolute risk for progression at 20 y (%)	Absolute risk for progression at 20 y accounting for death as a competing risk (%)
High risk stratification model incorporating all three predictive factors				
Low risk (serum M protein <1.5 g/dL, IgG subtype, normal free light chain ratio [0.26–1.65])	449	1	5	2
Low–intermediate risk (any one factor abnormal)	420	5.4	21	10
High–intermediate risk (any two factors abnormal)	226	10.1	37	18
High risk (all three factors abnormal)	53	20.8	58	27

(*Adapted from* Rajkumar SV, Kyle RA, Therneau TM, et al. Serum free light chain ratio
is an independent risk factor for progression in monoclonal gammopathy of undetermined significance. Blood 2005;106(3):812–7; with permission. © The American Society of Hematology.)

clinical deterioration of the neuropathy despite treatment, re-evaluation for
underlying malignant lymphoproliferative disorders or amyloidosis is pru-
dent [5].

Smoldering multiple myeloma and multiple myeloma

Smoldering multiple myeloma (SMM) accounts for 15% of all cases of
newly diagnosed MM. Similarly to MGUS, SMM is classified as an asymptomatic premalignant condition. MGUS and SMM are distinguished from
each other based on the size of the serum M protein and bone marrow
plasma cell percentage. Unlike MGUS the risk for progression to MM is
much higher in SMM: 1% in MGUS versus 10% to 20% in SMM. Most
patients who have SMM progress to MM in 3 to 4 years with some variability [23]. Treatment for SMM like MGUS is observation alone but with more
frequent follow-up, typically every 3 to 4 months [24].

MM is distinguished by the propagation of a single clone of plasma cells
engaged in the production of a specific immunoglobulin. MM evolves from

a premalignant state of MGUS through unknown mechanisms. This neo-plastic process occurs in the bone marrow and invades adjacent bone, caus-ing skeletal destruction [24]. Bone pain (particularly in the back or chest), weakness, pallor, and fatigue are the typical presenting clinical features. Renal insufficiency, hypercalcemia, and anemia are other key clinical flags. Organ involvement includes the kidneys, less commonly the liver, and in-creased propensity for neurologic involvement, most often in the form of compression of adjacent neural structures. Neurologic complications are usually related to compression of the spinal cord or roots from lytic verte-bral lesions, and symptoms are localized [25]. Peripheral neuropathy associ-ated with MM is rare, occurring in approximately 5% of patients and usually presenting as a distal sensorimotor polyneuropathy. Nerve conduc-tion studies and sural nerve biopsy are typically consistent with an axonal process with loss of myelinated fibers [25].

The incidence of MM is approximately 4 per 100,000 per year, accounting for 1% of all malignant disease [26]. Diagnostic criteria for MM includes the presence of bone marrow plasma cells greater than or equal to 10%, presence of M-protein, and evidence of lytic bone lesions or other underlying organ failure that can be attributed to an underlying plasma cell disorder (see Table 2). Because AL amyloidosis complicates MM in 30% to 40% of cases, it is recommended that patients who have MM have tissue or nerve biopsy per-formed to identify amyloidosis. Treatment of patients who have MM consists of radiation therapy, chemotherapy, autologous peripheral stem cell trans-plantation with conventional therapy, and novel targeted research trials [27].

Variant forms of multiple myeloma

Solitary plasmacytoma

Solitary plasmacytoma (SP) may be confined to bone or may arise in extra-medullary sites. There are a few reports of an association between solitary myelomas and peripheral neuropathy [21]. The presence of biopsy-proven solitary lesion of bone or tissue with evidence of clonal plasma cells and the absence of end organ damage is suggestive of plasmacytoma (see further diagnostic criteria in Table 2). An MRI scan of the spine and pelvis should be performed in addition to a skeletal survey, because one third of patients who have SP may have additional occult lesions. Surgical removal and irra-diation of the involved site is the treatment of choice. Follow-up with close surveillance is mandatory because of the increased risk for full blown MM [6].

Polyneuropathy, organomegaly, endocrinopathy, monoclonal gammopathy, and skin changes syndrome

This is a rare atypical plasma cell proliferative disorder that can present as single or multiple plasmacytomas with one or more osteosclerotic lesions. The syndrome is important to recognize among the plasma cell disorders because it is treatable. The more common acronym POEMS is used to describe major clinical manifestations of the syndrome. Variable additional key features, however, including Castleman disease (giant lymph node hyperplasia, angiofollicular lymph node hyperplasia), papilledema, peripheral edema, ascites, polycythemia, thrombocytosis, and fatigue and clubbing are not included in the acronym. POEMS syndrome has been referred to as osteosclerotic myeloma, Crow-Fukase syndrome, PEP (*p*lasma cell dyscrasias, *e*ndocrinopathy, and *p*olyneuropathy) syndrome, and Takatsuki syndrome [28].

Although POEMS syndrome occurs in approximately 2% of patients who have MM, this neuropathy differs from that associated with MM in several aspects. Occurring at an earlier age (median age of 51 years), more commonly in men, POEMS neuropathy is more frequently a demyelinating, predominantly motor neuropathy with slowed motor nerve conduction velocities and elevated CSF protein levels. An M protein is found in 90% of cases, most often composed of λ light chains associated with IgG and IgA heavy chains. Approximately 85% of these patients present with a peripheral neuropathy that bears a striking resemblance to CIDP with symmetric proximal and distal weakness and variable sensory loss. The clinical and electrophysiologic similarities between CIDP and POEMS reinforce the importance of M-protein screening on all patients presenting with acquired demyelinating neuropathy [28].

Additional clinical features include sclerotic bone lesions (primarily in the axial skeleton), a varying spectrum of the aforementioned associated clinical abnormalities, and respiratory problems. The pathogenesis is unclear but may at least in part be cytokine-mediated with elevated vascular endothelial growth factor levels. The clinical course may vary from indolent to fulminating. Focused radiation therapy to the sclerotic lesions produces substantial improvement of clinical symptoms in more than 50% of patients in the dosage range of 40 to 50 cGy, with half of the patients showing improvement in their neuropathy symptoms. Unlike in CIDP, plasmapheresis and intravenous immunoglobulin do not reliably show clinical benefit. For widespread involvement, autologous stem cell transplantation has proved helpful, as has chemotherapy with mephalan and prednisone [29].

Waldenström macroglobulinemia

Waldenström macroglobulinemia (WM) is the consequence of uncontrolled malignant proliferation of lymphocytes and plasma cells that secrete large quantities of monoclonal protein IgM. This condition is nearly 10% to 20% as common as MM and affects males slightly more often than females. The median age of onset is 65 years, with a preponderance of Caucasians more affected than African Americans. Presenting clinical symptoms include weakness, fatigue, and symptoms of hyperviscosity syndrome (oronasal bleeding, blurred vision, dizziness, and dyspnea) [30].

Approximately one third of patients who have WM have symptoms of peripheral neuropathy [31]. The typical neurologic presentation is chronic symmetric predominantly sensory polyneuropathy similar to the neuropathy associated with MGUS. Pure sensory polyneuropathy, multiple mononeuropathies, and painful predominately sensory neuropathy with prominent dysautonomia often associated with disordered gait are other clinical presentations. The central nervous system is rarely affected. When IgM binds to MAG or sulfatide there is an associated increase in the frequency and severity of peripheral nerve involvement [31]. In approximately half of this group of patients, nerve conduction studies show slowed motor nerve conduction velocities and prolonged distal latencies consistent with demyelinating neuropathy.

The serum protein electrophoresis shows an IgM monoclonal spike of greater than or equal to 3 g/dL, with 75% of these proteins having κ light chain. Reduced IgG and IgA protein titers are often associated. A small monoclonal light chain is found in the urine of most patients. The diagnosis of WM requires evidence of bone marrow infiltration by lymphoplasmacytoid lymphoma with the detection of serum IgM monoclonal protein (see Table 2). The bone marrow aspirate is hypocellular, but biopsy specimens are hypercellular with an increase in lymphocytes and plasma cells. Most patients have a moderate to severe normocytic, normochromic anemia. Nerve biopsy findings are similar to those seen in IgM MGUS [6,7,15].

The reported median survival for WM is approximately 5 years. Age older than 70 years, hemoglobin level less than 9 g/dL, weight loss, and cryoglobulinemia, however, are adverse predictive factors [6]. The asymptomatic patient without evidence of end organ damage is considered to have smoldering Waldenström macroglobulinemia, and immediate therapy is not required [15]. Anemia or thrombocytopenia and constitutional symptoms related to Waldenström macroglobulinemia are considered indications for therapy. Rituximab, nucleoside analogs, alkylating agents alone or rituximab in combination with nucleoside analogs, nucleoside analogs plus alkylating agents, and combination chemotherapy are the current treatment options for WM. Therapy is decided based on the age of the patient and the aggressiveness of the presentation. Because no randomized data exist to determine the best option, patients are preferably treated in clinical trials [6,32].

Systemic AL amyloidosis

Amyloidosis is a multisystem disorder characterized by extracellular deposition of fibrillar proteins that can be deposited in various organs and tissues throughout the body. Diagnosis is based on the recognition of amyloid deposits in the affected organs (Table 4) [6]. Amyloid can be detected when tissue is stained with Congo red dye, which displays a characteristic apple-green birefringence under polarized light and a characteristic ultrastructural

Table 4
Classification of amyloidosis

Types of amyloidosis	Major protein component	Clinical presentation
AL amyloidosis[a]	K or λ light chains	Primary or localized; polyneuropathy, autonomic dysfunction, rarely myopathy, nephrotic syndrome, cardiac failure, diarrheas, hypoalbuminemia, cutaneous purpura, macroglossia, and hepatomegaly
AA amyloidosis	Serum amyloid A protein	Chronic inflammatory conditions; typically acquired but hereditary in case of familial Mediterranean fever; renal presentation most common
ATTR amyloidosis		
Mutant TTR[b]	Mutated transthyretin	Hereditary: peripheral neuropathy and cardiomyopathy
Normal TTR (senile amyloidosis)	Normal transthyretin	Restrictive cardiomyopathy; carpal tunnel
B2-microglobulin amyloidosis	B2-microglobulin	Carpal tunnel
Aβ amyloidosis	Aβ protein precursor	Alzheimer syndrome
Other hereditary amyloidosis		
A fibrinogen (also called familial renal amyloidosis)	Fibrinogen α-chain	Renal presentation
Lysozyme	Lysozyme	Renal presentation most common
Apolipoprotein A-I	Apolipoprotein A-I	Renal presentation most common

[a] AL amyloidosis is the only form of amyloidosis that is secondary to a clonal plasma cell disorder. AL amyloidosis can be associated with multiple myeloma in approximately 10% of patients.

[b] TTR refers to transthyretin, which is commonly referred to as prealbumin.

(*Adapted from* Rajkumar SV, Dispenzieri A, Kyle RA. Monoclonal gammopathy of undetermined significance, Waldenström macroglobulinemia, AL amyloidosis, and related plasma cell disorders: diagnosis and treatment. Mayo Clin Proc 2006;81(5):693–703; with permission.)

appearance when examined under electron microscopy. The use of the protein composition of the amyloid material has allowed for classification of several distinct types of amyloidosis (Table 4) that may be localized or systemic [6]. Systemic AL amyloidosis is referred to as primary systemic amyloidosis or primary amyloidosis. AL (immunoglobulin light chain) amyloidosis refers to the type of amyloidosis resulting from the amino-terminus variable segment of immunoglobulin light chain. This variety commonly presents in the absence of a malignant plasma cell dyscrasia but may occur in association with MM or Waldenström macroglobulinemia. The pathogenesis of AL amyloidosis is poorly understood, but one hypothesis is uncontrolled expansion of a clone of either malignant or nonproliferative plasma cells that secrete amyloidogenic light chain polypeptides [33].

AL amyloidosis typically presents with polyneuropathy, autonomic symptoms, and much less often with proximal muscle weakness. More than half of the patients have systemic organ involvement (nephrotic syndrome, cardiac failure, chronic diarrhea with wasting, hypoalbuminemia, cutaneous purpura, macroglossia, and hepatomegaly) [33].

Peripheral neuropathy occurs in 15% to 30% of patients who have AL amyloidosis and is the presenting feature in 10% of the cases. The neuropathy has a slow, painful, distal progressive course. Loss of small fiber modalities is initially seen, with loss of light touch or vibratory sensation following, and most patients go on to develop autonomic dysfunction. Carpal tunnel syndrome caused by amyloid infiltration of the flexor retinaculum at the wrist occurs in approximately 25% of patients. Electrodiagnostic studies are consistent with axonal neuropathy. Nerve conduction studies show low amplitude to absent sensory nerve action potential, low amplitude, compound muscle action potentials, but preserved motor conduction velocities. Distal motor latencies are normal. Needle examination frequently provides evidence of active denervation.

Amyloid myopathy is rare and more often associated with AL type than familial amyloidosis. It is often overlooked, although there are clinical clues that include progressive proximal limb weakness, macroglossia, skeletal muscle hypertrophy, and palpable abnormality within muscle tissue and associated polyneuropathy symptoms [34,35]. The frequency of making the diagnosis of amyloid myopathy increases with the addition of Congo red and methyl violet staining of muscle biopsy specimens. Although amyloid myopathy is uncommon it should be considered in patients who have proximal weakness of uncertain cause [35].

The clinical prognosis is poor, with approximately 80% of patients succumbing within 36 months of diagnosis and approximately 50% with 12 months. Because mortality is primarily caused by cardiac failure, those patients who do not have cardiac and renal involvement have a better prognosis [36].

Mephalan and prednisone have been the mainstay of therapy, with unsatisfactory results. Stem cell transplantation is offered to some eligible patients, as are novel trials with thalidomide [36].

Miscellaneous disorders

Lower motor neuron syndromes

Multifocal motor neuropathy (MMN) is another lower motor neuron syndrome associated with increased titers of serum IgM autoantibodies to the ganglioside GM1 and to a lesser extent to other glycolipids. It is distinguished by its characteristic clinical picture, specific electrodiagnostic abnormalities, and frequently favorable response to IVIg. Patients typically present with a slowly progressive, predominantly distal asymmetric limb weakness and wasting, primarily in the arms. Deep tendon reflexes may be preserved early in the course of disease. Nerve conduction studies show evidence of multifocal motor conduction block (defined as a reduction of amplitude of 50% or more at proximal compared with distal sites of stimulation) in one or more nerves. The disorder is confined to motor axons with sparing of sensory axons [37]. The presence of antiGM1 antibodies is the most typical laboratory finding associated with MMN, although the proportion of affected patients who have the antibodies varies from 30% to 80%, and the degree of titer elevation ranges as markedly [38,39]. A rare condition affecting 1 to 2 persons per 100,000, MMN occurs more frequently in men than women and has a mean age of onset of approximately 40 years of age [27]. The effectiveness of IVIg therapy has been demonstrated in several studies and is widely considered the gold standard of treatment for MMN [36]. It is interesting that even after salutary treatment responses, the antiglycolipid levels often remain unchanged. This observation raises questions regarding the pathogenic role these antibodies play in MMN [28].

In the mid 1990s a subset of patients were identified who had purely axonal motor neuropathy with raised anti-GM1 antibody titers but no conduction block or other features suggesting demyelination and variable response to immunosuppressive therapy. The term multifocal acquired motor axonopathy (MAMA) was proposed for this group of patients [27]. An axonal NCS pattern, spontaneous activity, and chronic neurogenic motor unit potential changes in limb muscles, normal paraspinal muscle EMG, and increased anti-GD1 antibody titers were found in the group responsive to IVIg therapy [27].

Because of immunocytochemical studies showing binding of anti-ganglioside antibodies antigens on motor neuron cell bodies, axons at nodes of Ranvier and motor endplates, an association between MAMA and motor neuron disease has been raised. Although cases of high titers of IgM and anti-GM1 ganglioside antibodies have been reported in this disorder, there is little evidence of a causal link [4].

Cryoglobulinemia

Proteins (IgG or IgM) that precipitate when cooled, redissolve after warming, and circulate as immune complexes in the bloodstream are known as cryoglobulins. The immunoglobulin may be monoclonal or polyclonal or both. Cryoglobulinemia is divided into three types based on the composition of the cryoprecipitate: type 1, isolated monoclonal immunoglobulins; type II, a monoclonal mixture of an M-protein and polyclonal immunoglobulins (IgG) in the setting of lymphoproliferative disease or hepatitis C; and type III, polyclonal immunoglobulins in the setting of a collage-vascular or chronic inflammatory disease [5]. Cryoglobulinemia classically presents with purpura, arthralgias, asthenia, renal disease, and neuropathy. The disorder has most often been associated with hepatitis C, with less common associations including lymphoproliferative disorders, connective tissue disease, and other chronic infections. Peripheral neuropathy is reported in 17% to 56% of patients. This neuropathy may appear as either an acute or a subacute distal symmetric or asymmetric sensorimotor polyneuropathy or as mononeuropathy multiplex. Sensory symptoms usually precede motor manifestations. Most often an axonal pathophysiology predominates, although evidence suggesting demyelination may be present [40].

The therapeutic approach to mildly symptomatic cryoglobulinemia consists of conservative measures, such as bed rest, avoidance of cold, use of analgesics, and consideration of low-dose steroids. For more severe forms complicated by glomerulonephritis, motor neuropathy, and systemic vasculitis, plasmapheresis, high-dose steroids, and cytotoxic therapy may be warranted. The potential benefits of agents such as melphalan, cyclophosphamide, or chlorambucil must be weighed against the risk for myelodysplastic syndromes or acute leukemia. Interferon has been reported to be of benefit to those patients who have hepatitis C, although most relapse 6 months after discontinuation of this agent. Although purpuric lesions and liver function abnormalities show a rapid response, the neuropathy and nephropathy are slower to improve. Rituximab has recently been suggested as an alternative to traditional chemotherapy [5].

Summary

The last 2 decades have seen increased recognition of the clinical importance of peripheral neuropathies associated with monoclonal proteins. At least 10% of de novo neuropathy patients have an M protein. Despite that the discovery of an associated serious or frankly malignant disease, such as MM, Waldenström macroglobulinemia, POEMS, lymphoma, and AL amyloidosis, is uncommon in this group, these individuals require investigation for an underlying cause. Most are ultimately designated as having MGUS. The evaluation of paraproteinemias includes recognition of the M-protein through various biochemical studies and through performing additional testing, including a skeletal survey and aspirated bone marrow biopsy. Because the 25-year risk for progression to myeloma in MGUS is 30%, a recommendation for annual follow-up with measurement of total protein concentration and electrophoresis of serum and urine seems appropriate. Although no treatment is indicated for mild or subclinical MGUS, research in the arena of neoplastic plasma cell diseases has led to new therapies, including stem cell transplantation. Innovative research protocols are underway at several centers. Recognition of the syndromes associated with monoclonal gammopathies and peripheral neuropathy is essential for clinicians caring for these patients, as is familiarity with treatment options that may prove to be beneficial for many selected individuals.

References

[1] Kyle RA, Therneau TM, Rajkumar SV, et al. Long-term follow-up of 241 patients with monoclonal gammopathy of undetermined significance: the original Mayo Clinic series 25 years later. Mayo Clin Proc 2004;79(7):859–66.

[2] Landgren O, Gridley G, Turesson I, et al. Risk of monoclonal gammopathy of undetermined significance (MGUS) and subsequent multiple myeloma among African American and white veterans in the United States. Blood 2006;107(3):904–6.

[3] Kyle RA, Rajkumar SV. Plasma cell disorders. In: Goldman L, Ausiello D, editors. Cecil textbook of medicine, vol. 1. 22nd edition. Philadelphia: Saunders; 2004. p. 1184–95.

[4] Kyle RA, Dyck PK. Neuropathy associated with monoclonal gammopathies. In: Dyck PJ, Thomas PK, editors. Peripheral Neuropathy vol. 2. 4th edition. Philadelphia: Elsevier Saunders; 2005. p. 2255–2276.

[5] Dispenzieri A, Kyle RA. Neurological aspects of multiple myeloma and related disorders. Best Pract Res Clin Haematol 2005;18(4):673–88.

[6] Kyle RA, Rajkumar SV. Monoclonal gammopathies of undetermined significance. Rev Clin Exp Hematol 2002;6(3):225–52.

[7] Kyle RA, Rajkumar SV. Monoclonal gammopathies of undetermined significance: a review. Immunol Rev 2003;194:112–39.

[8] Quarles RH, Weiss MD. Autoantibodies associated with peripheral neuropathy. Muscle Nerve 1999;22(7):800–22.

[9] Kyle RA, Rajkumar SV. Multiple myeloma. N Engl J Med 2004;351(18):1860–73.

[10] Latov N, Hays AP, Sherman WH. Peripheral neuropathy and anti-MAG antibodies. Crit Rev Neurobiol 1988;3(4):301–32.

[11] Chassande B, Leger JM, Younes-Chennoufi AB, et al. Peripheral neuropathy associated with IgM monoclonal gammopathy: correlations between M-protein antibody activity and clinical/electrophysiological features in 40 cases. Muscle Nerve 1998;21(1):55–62.

[12] Roodman GD. Role of the bone marrow microenvironment in multiple myeloma. J Bone Miner Res 2002;17(11):1921–5.

[13] Gosselin S, Kyle RA, Dyck PJ. Neuropathy associated with monoclonal gammopathies of undetermined significance. Ann Neurol 1991;30(1):54–61.

[14] Yeung KB, Thomas PK, King RH, et al. The clinical spectrum of peripheral neuropathies associated with benign monoclonal IgM, IgG and IgA paraproteinaemia. Comparative clinical, immunological and nerve biopsy findings. J Neurol 1991;238(7):383–91.

[15] Blade J. Clinical practice. Monoclonal gammopathy of undetermined significance. N Engl J Med 2006;355(26):2765–70.

[16] Katzmann JA, Dispenzieri A, Kyle RA, et al. Elimination of the need for urine studies in the screening algorithm for monoclonal gammopathies by using serum immunofixation and free light chain assays. Mayo Clin Proc 2006;81(12):1575–8.

[17] Rajkumar SV, Dispenzieri A, Kyle RA. Monoclonal gammopathy of undetermined significance, Waldenstrom macroglobulinemia, AL amyloidosis, and related plasma cell disorders: diagnosis and treatment. Mayo Clin Proc 2006;81(5):693–703.

[18] Kyle RA, Therneau TM, Rajkumar SV, et al. Prevalence of monoclonal gammopathy of undetermined significance. N Engl J Med 2006;354(13):1362–9.

[19] Kyle RA, Rajkumar SV. Monoclonal gammopathy of undetermined significance. Br J Haematol 2006;134(6):573–89.

[20] Kissel JT, Mendell JR. Neuropathies associated with monoclonal gammopathies. Neuromuscul Disord 1996;6(1):3–18.

[21] Kyle RA, Dispenzieri A. Neuropathy associated with the monoclonal gammopathies. In: Noseworthy JH, editor. Neurological therapeutics principles and practice, vol. 3. 2nd edition. Abingdon, Oxon (UK): Informa Healthcare; 2006. p. 2401–14.

[22] Rajkumar SV, Kyle RA, Therneau TM, et al. Serum free light chain ratio is an independent risk factor for progression in monoclonal gammopathy of undetermined significance. Blood 2005;106(3):812–7.

[23] Rajkumar SV. MGUS and smoldering multiple myeloma: update on pathogenesis, natural history, and management. Hematology Am Soc Hematol Educ Program 2005;340–5.

[24] Blade J, Rosinol L. Smoldering multiple myeloma and monoclonal gammopathy of undetermined significance. Curr Treat Options Oncol 2006;7(3):237–45.

[25] Sirohi B, Powles R. Multiple myeloma. Lancet 2004;363(9412):875–87.

[26] Kyle RA, Gertz MA, Witzig TE, et al. Review of 1027 patients with newly diagnosed multiple myeloma. Mayo Clin Proc 2003;78(1):21–33.

[27] Rajkumar SV, Kyle RA. Multiple myeloma: diagnosis and treatment. Mayo Clin Proc 2005; 80(10):1371–82.

[28] Dispenzieri A, Kyle RA. Multiple myeloma: clinical features and indications for therapy. Best Pract Res Clin Haematol 2005;18(4):553–68.

[29] Dispenzieri A, Moreno-Aspitia A, Suarez GA, et al. Peripheral blood stem cell transplantation in 16 patients with POEMS syndrome, and a review of the literature. Blood 2004; 104(10):3400–7.

[30] Dimopoulos MA, Kyle RA, Anagnostopoulos A, et al. Diagnosis and management of Waldenström's macroglobulinemia. J Clin Oncol 2005;23(7):1564–77.

[31] Levine T, Pestronk A, Florence J, et al. Peripheral neuropathies in Waldenström's macroglobulinaemia. J Neurol Neurosurg Psychiatry 2006;77(2):224–8.

[32] Treon SP, Gertz MA, Dimopoulos M, et al. Update on treatment recommendations from the Third International Workshop on Waldenström's macroglobulinemia. Blood 2006;107(9): 3442–6.

[33] Kyle RA, Kelly JJ, Dyck PJ. Amyloidosis and neuropathy peripheral neuropathy, vol. 2. Philadelphia: Elsevier Saunders; 2005. p. 2427–51.

[34] Spuler S, Emslie-Smith A, Engel AG. Amyloid myopathy: an underdiagnosed entity. Ann Neurol 1998;43(6):719–28.

[35] Chapin JE, Kornfeld M, Harris A. Amyloid myopathy: characteristic features of a still underdiagnosed disease. Muscle Nerve 2005;31(2):266–72.

[36] Gertz MA, Kyle RA. Amyloidosis with IgM monoclonal gammopathies. Semin Oncol 2003; 30(2):325–8.

[37] Bosch EP, Smith BE. Peripheral neuropathies associated with monoclonal proteins. Med Clin North Am 1993;77(1):125–39.

[38] Leger JM, Behin A. Multifocal motor neuropathy. Curr Opin Neurol 2005;18(5):567–73.

[39] Parry GJ. Antiganglioside antibodies do not necessarily play a role in multifocal motor neuropathy. Muscle Nerve 1994;17(1):97–9.

[40] Ropper AH, Gorson KC. Neuropathies associated with paraproteinemia. N Engl J Med 1998;338(22):1601–7.

ELSEVIER
SAUNDERS

Phys Med Rehabil Clin N Am
19 (2008) 81–96

PHYSICAL MEDICINE
AND REHABILITATION
CLINICS OF
NORTH AMERICA

Neuromuscular Complications of Human Immunodeficiency Virus Infection

Jessica Robinson-Papp, MD*, David M. Simpson, MD

*Department of Neurology, Mount Sinai Medical Center,
Box 1052, New York, NY 10029, USA*

Advances in the treatment of HIV with highly active antiretroviral therapy have led to improved longevity and overall health in patients living with HIV. Prolonged lifespan results in increased cumulative exposure to the HIV virus, associated infectious agents, and potentially neurotoxic therapies, and provides increased opportunity for chronic neurologic conditions to develop. HIV affects both the central and peripheral nervous systems and different lesions may coexist in a single patient. HIV-positive patients may also develop neurologic disease unrelated to HIV. This article describes the complications of HIV in the peripheral nervous system (PNS) and muscle, summarized in Table 1. Because of the potential for multiple lesions, the approach to an HIV-positive patient presenting with neurologic symptoms must be comprehensive. The evaluation begins with a detailed history and general physical and neurologic examination, which leads to neuroanatomic localization and differential diagnosis.

The PNS can be divided into somatic and autonomic systems, and further subdivided into motor and sensory systems. The somatic motor neurons arise in the anterior horn of the spinal cord, exit the spinal cord as the ventral nerve root, then join with sensory fibers, originating in the dorsal root ganglion to form nerve plexus and peripheral nerve. The motor axon terminates at the neuromuscular junction where it innervates muscle. Autonomic efferents arise in the brain stem and the intermediolateral cell column of the spinal cord, travel to sympathetic and parasympathetic ganglia, and ultimately to their target organs.

---

* Corresponding author.
E-mail address: jessica.robinson-papp@mssm.edu (J. Robinson-Papp).

1047-9651/08/$ - see front matter
doi:10.1016/j.pmr.2007.10.009

ROBINSON-PAPP & SIMPSON

Table 1
Summary of neuromuscular complications of HIV

Disease	Time of onset	Incidence	Clinical features	Prognosis	Treatment
Distal sensory polyneuropathy	May be more common in advanced HIV	Common: 30%–58% of patients	Sensory loss, pain, and parasthesias beginning in feet	Chronic; pain can significantly interfere with quality of life	Withdrawal of neurotoxic agents Pain management: TCAs, SNRIs, AEDs, topical therapies
Autonomic neuropathy	Any time in disease course	Common, but usually subclinical	Orthostatic hypotension, syncope, cardiac arrhythmias, diarrhea, erectile and urinary dysfunction	Chronic; symptoms may reduce quality of life	Symptomatic for orthostasis; cardiology consult for suspected arrhythmia
Inflammatory demyelinating polyneuropathy	Seroconversion or early or late HIV	Rare	Ascending weakness; parasthesias	Good; major recovery within 4 weeks typical, full recovery more protracted	IVIg, plasmapheresis; corticosteroids for CIDP Late: Ganciclovir, foscarnet, cidofovir
HIV-associated neuromuscular weakness syndrome	Any time in disease course	Rare	Rapidly progressive weakness nausea, vomiting, weight loss, abdominal pain, hepatomegaly	Variable. Significant mortality, some patients with full recovery	Withdrawal of NRTI IVIg, plasmapheresis, corticosteroids; supportive care

Mononeuropathy multiplex	Early and late forms	Rare	Early: sensorimotor deficits in 1–2 nerves Late: many nerves involved	Early: good; usually self-limited Late: poorer; may not recover fully	Early: no treatment or corticosteroids, IVIg, plasmapheresis Late: ganciclovir, foscarnet, cidofovir
Progressive poly-radiculopathy	Advanced infection	Rare	Rapid onset, flaccid paraparesis	Poor; high mortality if untreated; incomplete recovery common	Ganciclovir, foscarnet, cidofovir
Myopathy	Any stage	Moderate	Slowly, progressive proximal weakness	Fair; course slow, may improve with treatment	ZDV/NRTI withdrawal; corticosteroids, IVIg

Abbreviations: AED, antiepileptic drugs; CIDP, chronic inflammatory demyelinating polyneuropathy; IVIg, intravenous immunoglobulin; NRTI, nucleoside analog reverse transcriptase inhibitors; SNRI, serotonin-norepinephrine reuptake inhibitors; TCA, tricyclic antidepressants; ZDV, zidovudine.

Disease processes may affect any of these neural elements. The pattern of deficits described by the patient and found on neurologic examination, provide clues to the localization, which in turn guides differential diagnosis. For example, in the absence of sensory symptoms, pure motor weakness, usually symmetric and more prominent proximally, suggests a lesion affecting the muscle or neuromuscular junction. Distal, symmetric sensory symptoms are seen in HIV-related polyneuropathies. Motor and sensory symptoms occur together focally in mononeuropathy multiplex, and more diffusely in acute inflammatory demyelinating polyneuropathy (AIDP) and progressive polyradiculopathy. The suspected localization of the lesion assists in guiding further evaluation, including laboratory, neuroimaging, and neurophysiologic studies, and ultimately leads to diagnosis, patient counseling, and a management strategy.

Neuropathies and radiculopathies

The primary components of peripheral nerves are motor and sensory axons and myelin. The motor axon is a projection of the anterior horn cell body, located in the spinal cord. The sensory axon takes its origin from the dorsal root ganglion, which also sends a projection to the spinal cord via the dorsal root. Myelin is produced by Schwann cells, and envelops many of the axons to provide the electrical insulation that permits rapid signal conduction. Neuropathies may result from damage either to the axon itself or to the myelin sheath. Radiculopathies occur when nerve roots are compromised, and may involve damage to both the myelin and axons.

Distal sensory polyneuropathy

Distal sensory polyneuropathy (DSP) is the most common neurologic complication of HIV, and may be present in 50% or more of patients with advanced disease. Although classically thought of as a feature of advanced HIV, DSP may also occur in patients with good immunologic status and virologic control [1]. Recent cohort studies indicate that the primary risk factor for DSP is advancing age, and that CD4 count and HIV plasma viral load are no longer predictive [2].

Clinical features

Symptoms of DSP include pain, burning, and numbness. Patients may also experience allodynia, defined as pain caused by innocuous stimuli, such as light touch. Symptoms begin in a distal symmetric distribution, typically affecting the toes and soles of the feet first. As the neuropathy progresses, the distal legs, and ultimately fingers and hands, may become involved. Weakness is not a common early feature of DSP; however, in severe cases the muscles of the feet may be mildly weak.

Neurologic examination typically reveals diminished sense of temperature, pain, and vibration in a distal distribution. Proprioception is relatively spared. Ankle reflexes are diminished or absent. Reflexes at the knees are usually normal, or may even be hyperactive because of coexisting central nervous system disease. Weakness of the intrinsic muscles of the feet is assessed by asking the patient to curl the toes down, dorsiflex, or separate them. Loss of hair and tightness of the skin in the calves may be seen on general physical examination.

Pathogenesis

DSP is a length-dependent process resulting from damage to the most distal segments of the sensory axon. Small myelinated and unmyelinated fibers are typically the first affected; thus, DSP is often referred to as a "small fiber neuropathy." DSP may occur as a result of HIV itself, or as a side effect of neurotoxic antiretroviral (ARV) therapy. There is no evidence for direct infection of axons or Schwann cells by the HIV virus, and the mechanism by which HIV causes axonal damage is likely caused by secondary factors, such as immune-mediated neurotoxicity. HIV-induced dysregulation of macrophages and overproduction of inflammatory cytokines is one possible mechanism [3]. Schwann-cell mediated neurotoxicity caused by an HIV-associated glycoprotein, gp120, has also been proposed [4]. ARV-associated DSP occurs most commonly in patients treated with the nucleoside analog reverse transcriptase inhibitors (NRTI) didanosine (ddI), zalcitarabine (ddC), and stavudine (d4T). These agents, commonly referred to as "d-drugs," appear to cause mitochondrial toxicity [5]. There is emerging evidence that several drugs of the protease inhibitor class—namely indinavir, saquinavir, and ritonavir—may also be associated with neuropathy [6].

Diagnostic testing

Although DSP in the HIV-positive patient is most often related to HIV infection or ARV toxicity, it is important to determine whether the patient has other risk factors for neuropathy, such as alcohol abuse, poor nutritional status, diabetes mellitus, autoimmune disease, malignancy, or dysfunction of the kidney, liver, or thyroid. Diagnostic studies should include blood tests, such as a complete metabolic panel, liver function tests, hemoglobin A1c, vitamin B_{12} level, thyroid function tests, venereal disease research laboratory, hepatitis serology, erythrocyte sedimentation rate, antinuclear antibody, and serum protein electrophoresis.

DSP is primarily a clinical diagnosis and further diagnostic procedures may not be necessary. In atypical cases, nerve conduction studies (NCS) and electromyography (EMG) may be helpful; however, a normal result does not exclude DSP, as NCS and EMG have a low sensitivity for the detection of small fiber neuropathy. When abnormalities are seen, decreased or absent sensory nerve action potentials in the distal lower extremity are typically the earliest findings. In more advanced cases, motor conduction studies and late responses may be abnormal, and EMG may show denervation in distal muscles.

There has been increasing interest in the use of epidermal skin biopsy in the diagnosis of DSP [7]. In this technique, a sample of skin is obtained by punch biopsy from a distal and proximal site in the lower extremity. The epidermal nerve fiber density is then determined and compared with standardized values. As small fiber neuropathies are difficult to detect by conventional studies, reduced epidermal nerve fiber density may be the only abnormal diagnostic result.

Therapy

Treatment of DSP is largely symptomatic, as there are currently no neuroregenerative agents available. Any reversible causes of neuropathy identified during the diagnostic evaluation should be addressed, especially discontinuation of any neurotoxic medications when possible. Of note, DSP secondary to ARV may persist and even worsen for several weeks after cessation of the offending medication, a phenomenon termed "coasting syndrome" [8].

Symptomatic treatment of DSP focuses on management of the positive symptoms of neuropathy, such as pain and paresthesias. There are no specific treatments for the negative symptoms, such as numbness, ataxia, and weakness, other than rehabilitation therapy. Before beginning treatment, and at each visit throughout the course of treatment, the patient's pain level should be systematically documented. Pain scales are helpful for quantifying the patient's pain. A numeric pain intensity scale is commonly used in adults and rates pain on a scale from 0 to 10, where 0 is no pain and 10 is the worst possible pain. The pain intensity scale can be used as part of a pain management flow sheet to document changes over time (Table 2). The degree of pain that the patient experiences and the frequency of pain throughout the day will guide the course of treatment.

There are limited clinical trials, and no Food and Drug Administration (FDA)-approved therapies for the treatment of HIV-associated DSP.

Table 2
Pain management flow sheet

Patient name:
Date:
What is your current pain level[a]?
What is the worst pain you have experienced in the last 24 hours[a]?
What percentage of the time do you experience your worst pain?
What is your average pain level[a]?
What percentage of the time are you pain free?

[a] Rated as 0 = no pain to 10 = worst possible pain.

However, there is extensive experience with medications used in an off-label fashion. For mild or intermittent discomfort it is reasonable to begin with an over-the-counter analgesic, such as acetaminophen, used as needed. For more chronic or severe pain, a standing pain management regimen with an additional agent used as needed for breakthrough pain, is more appropriate. For intractable pain, multiple agents used in combination may be needed. Medications used for the management of DSP fall into four main categories: antiepileptics, antidepressants, topical agents, and nonspecific analgesics (Table 3).

Nearly all of the newer antiepileptic drugs (AEDs) have been used in the treatment of neuropathic pain. Pregabalin provides analgesia by inhibiting the α-2-Δ presynaptic voltage gated calcium channels, and reducing calcium influx and the release of excitatory neurotransmitters associated with neuropathic pain [9]. Pregabalin is FDA-approved for the treatment of painful diabetic neuropathy [10]. Pregabalin is currently being studied in clinical trials for the treatment of HIV-associated DSP, but is already commonly used off-label.

Pregabalin is commonly initiated at 75 mg, twice a day, and may be increased to a maximum dose of 300 mg, twice a day. It is typically well tolerated, and the most common side effects, dizziness and somnolence, are frequently transient and minimized by beginning with a low dose. Pregabalin is metabolized and excreted by the kidney, which is advantageous in HIV-positive patients who are often taking hepatically metabolized ARV.

Gabapentin is an older compound with a similar mechanism of action, side effect profile, and metabolism to pregabalin. Gabapentin has been used extensively in clinical practice and was shown to be effective in reducing pain in HIV-associated DSP in one small placebo-controlled trial [11]. As with pregabalin, gabapentin is usually started at low doses, such as

Table 3
Summary of adjuvant treatment options for neuropathic pain

Drug	Dosage	Common side effects
Amitriptyline, other TCA	10 mg po qhs to start, titrate to efficacy	Sedation, confusion, orthostatic hypotension, urinary retention, dry mouth, and blurred vision
Duloxetine	30 mg po qd to start, increase to 60 mg po qd	Nausea, dizziness, somnolence, fatigue
Gabapentin	100 mg po tid to start, titrate to 800 mg–1,200 mg tid	Somnolence, dizziness, fatigue
Lamotrigine	25 mg po daily to start, slow titration to 200 mg bid to avoid rash	Rash, dizziness, ataxia, somnolence, headache
Lidocaine patch	Apply patch to affected area for 12–24 hours	Local irritation
Pregabalin	75 mg po bid to start, titrate to 150 mg–300 mg bid	Somnolence, dizziness

100 mg three times a day, although doses as large as 3,600 mg daily are often tolerated. Gabapentin is now available in a generic form. While there are no head-to-head comparison studies of gabapentin and pregabalin, pregabalin has linear pharmacokinetics, better bioavailability, and a more convenient titration schedule.

Among the other AEDs, lamotrigine has been found to be effective in HIV-DSP, but is used less frequently in clinical practice in part because of the potential side effect of rash, and a long titration schedule [12]. Zonisamide, topiramate, and oxcarbazepine have demonstrated some efficacy for painful diabetic neuropathy in clinical trials, but the role for these agents in the treatment of HIV-associated DSP is unclear [13–15].

Antidepressants, specifically the tricyclic antidepressants (TCAs) and the selective serotonin-norepinephrine reuptake inhibitors (SNRIs), are another major class of medications used in the treatment of DSP. TCAs inhibit the reuptake of numerous neurotransmitters, including monoamines and acetylcholine, while SNRIs are selective for serotonin and norepinepherine. These agents are thought to exert their analgesic effect via enhancement of central descending pain inhibition pathways.

Duloxetine, an SNRI, is FDA-approved for the treatment of diabetic neuropathic pain [16]. Although it has not been studied in the treatment of HIV-associated DSP, it is often used off-label. The most common side effect of duloxetine is nausea, which is usually transient. This symptom may be minimized by beginning duloxetine at a low dose, such as 20 mg to 30 mg daily, and titrating to the recommended and proven effective dose of 60 mg daily by the second week of treatment. The dose may be further increased to 90 mg to 120 mg daily if there is insufficient response. Duloxetine undergoes hepatic metabolism, and levels may be increased by medications that inhibit the 2D6 isozyme of cytochrome P450, such as tipranavir, ritonavir, and delavirdine [17]. Similarly, duloxetine inhibits 2D6 metabolism, and thus may increase serum levels of drugs that are 2D6 substrates, such as tricyclic antidepressants. Caution must also be exercised in combining duloxetine with other serotonergic drugs because of the risk of serotonin syndrome. Venlafaxine is another SNRI that has been studied for the treatment of neuropathic pain, particularly diabetic, although it is not FDA-approved for this indication.

TCAs have been available for over 50 years, and agents of this class, such as amitriptyline and nortriptyline, are still commonly used for neuropathic pain and other chronic pain syndromes. Although quite effective as neuropathic analgesics, the use of TCAs is commonly limited by side effects that include sedation, confusion, orthostatic hypotension, urinary retention, dry mouth, blurred vision, and cardiac arrythmia [18]. Starting with a single low evening dose, such as amitriptyline 10 mg to 25 mg, may improve tolerability. Nortriptyline typically has fewer side effects than amitriptyline. Like duloxetine, TCAs also undergo extensive hepatic metabolism via the cytochome P450, and therefore have potential for interaction with ARV.

Topical therapies are attractive for the treatment of DSP because the symptoms are often localized to a circumscribed area, and there is minimal potential for systemic side effects or interaction with oral medications. Topical lidocaine, in gel and patch form, has been used with limited success [19]. A high dose capsaicin patch was found to be safe and effective in controlled clinical trials of painful HIV DSP, but is not yet commercially available [20].

Antiepileptics, antidepressants, and topical treatments are all therapies which must be used regularly to provide around the clock analgesia, but are not useful in the treatment of acute pain. It is increasingly recognized that even patients whose pain is generally well controlled may experience acute exacerbations, termed "breakthrough pain" [21]. A model for treatment of chronic pain with a standing regimen, supplemented with additional fast-acting medications for breakthrough pain, was initially described by the World Health Organization for the treatment of cancer-related pain [22]. This model is now being explored in the treatment of neuropathic pain. A recent meta-analysis of opioids in the treatment of neuropathic pain showed efficacy of standing opioid therapy for chronic pain, and mixed results for the treatment of acute pain [23]. Recent studies support the safety and efficacy of a rapid-acting opioid, fentanyl buccal tablet in the treatment of neuropathic pain [24]. Further study of the clinical features and optimal treatment for neuropathic breakthrough pain is needed.

Autonomic neuropathy

Autonomic nerves are composed primarily of small myelinated and unmyelinated fibers, similar to the fibers most affected in DSP. While autonomic dysfunction is reported to be common in HIV infection, it is usually subclinical [25]. Symptoms of autonomic neuropathy are reported far less frequently than DSP, usually in the context of advanced HIV. Both sympathetic and parasympathetic systems are affected, and symptoms may include orthostatic hypotension, syncope, cardiac arrhythmias, anhidrosis, diarrhea, and erectile and urinary dysfunction. As in DSP, the precise mechanism of autonomic neuropathy is uncertain. Pathologic specimens show inflammatory infiltration of sympathetic ganglia. Both autoimmunity and direct infection by the HIV virus have been proposed as possible mechanisms [26].

Autonomic studies, such as tilt-table testing, may be helpful to confirm the diagnosis of autonomic neuropathy. Patients with a history suggestive of cardiac arrhythmia should be evaluated by a cardiologist. Initial management of orthostatic hypotension is conservative, and includes cessation of any medications associated with hypotension, increased salt and fluid intake, compressive stockings, and avoidance of the supine position. If conservative measures fail, medications such as midodrine and fludrocortisone may be tried.

Inflammatory demyelinating polyneuropathy

Acute inflammatory demyelinating polyneuropathy (AIDP), also known as Guillain-Barre syndrome, is a relatively uncommon complication of HIV. It is typically seen in the early stages of HIV and may be associated with seroconversion [27]. AIDP is caused by multifocal, immune-mediated demyelination of peripheral nerve. In some patients with AIDP in the setting of advanced immunosuppression, cytomegalovirus (CMV) has been demonstrated to be the causative organism [28].

AIDP in the setting of HIV is phenotypically similar to AIDP in the HIV-uninfected population. Patients present with rapidly progressive symmetric weakness, usually beginning in the distal lower extremities and ascending to involve the proximal lower extremities, upper extremities, and in severe cases, respiratory muscles. Although AIDP is a predominantly motor syndrome, pain and paresthesias in the back and legs may be a prominent early complaint.

Neurologic examination reveals diffuse weakness, usually more marked in the distal lower extremities, decreased or absent deep tendon reflexes, and relative sparing of sensation. Symmetric facial weakness is a relatively common and distinctive feature and can help distinguish AIDP from other causes of progressive weakness. The examiner may elicit facial weakness by asking the patient to close the eyes forcibly or to puff out the cheeks. If strength is normal, the examiner should be unable to open the patient's eyes and air should not escape through the lips if pressure is applied to the cheeks. Other cranial nerve abnormalities are unusual.

There are several variants of AIDP. Miller-Fisher syndrome is characterized by a triad of ophthalmoparesis, ataxia, and areflexia, and accounts for 5% to 10% of cases of AIDP in the general population, but is rarely reported in HIV-positive patients [29,30]. In the axonal variant of AIDP, axons, rather than myelin, are the primary target of autoimmunity. These patients present with a more severe and protracted course, and may have more marked involvement of the autonomic nervous system, leading to potentially life threatening fluctuations in heart rate and blood pressure. Chronic inflammatory demyelinating polyneuropathy (CIDP) has a more indolent course, and usually presents with weakness and numbness evolving over months, occasionally with a relapsing course.

AIDP is a neurologic emergency, as patients may deteriorate rapidly and develop respiratory insufficiency or autonomic instability. Accordingly, patients suspected of having AIDP are admitted to the hospital for continuous cardiovascular monitoring and regular pulmonary function tests. Diagnostic studies used to confirm the diagnosis include NCS and EMG, and lumbar puncture for cerebrospinal fluid examination.

While NCS in AIDP may show only mild abnormalities, evolving and chronic demyelination results in slowing of conduction along affected segments. When more marked, this may cause incomplete transmission of signals, known as conduction block. NCS reveals slowing of nerve conduction velocities, temporal dispersion, and prolongation of late responses and distal motor latencies. Conduction block will result in a loss of amplitude of the response across a demyelinated segment, and reduced recruitment on needle EMG.

Cerebrospinal fluid abnormalities seen in AIDP in HIV-positive patients include elevated protein level and a predominantly lymphocytic pleocytosis. This is distinctive from findings in HIV-negative patients, in whom increased protein levels occur without associated pleocytosis, so called cytoalbuminemic dissociation.

As there have been no controlled trials of the treatment of AIDP or CIDP in the setting of HIV, the management recommendations are derived from the literature of inflammatory demyelinating polyneuropathy (IDP) in the HIV-unifected population. AIDP and CIDP are generally treated with intravenous immunoglobulin (IVIg) or plasmaphoresis [31]. While corticosteroids are also effective in HIV-negative CIDP, they should be used with caution in HIV infection because of their immunosuppressive effects. For IDP occurring in patients with advanced immunosuppression, anti-CMV therapy may be used, especially if the presence of CMV in cerebrospinal fluid is documented, preferably with a polymerase chain reaction (PCR) assay. CMV inclusions can also be detected on nerve biopsy specimens. Comprehensive supportive care is also essential.

Detailed prognostic data for IDP in the HIV-positive population is not available, so patients must be counseled based on data from the general population. Specifically, patients should be aware that symptoms may continue to worsen, and be warned about the potential for respiratory compromise, requiring intubation. They should be advised that while most patients ultimately recover fully, complete recovery may take as long as 1 to 2 years, and incomplete recovery is more common in CIDP.

HIV-associated neuromuscular weakness syndrome

HIV-associated neuromuscular weakness syndrome (HANWS) presents with rapidly progressive weakness, clinically similar to AIDP [32]. Associated systemic symptoms include nausea, vomiting, weight loss, abdominal distention, hepatomegaly, and lipoatrophy. HANWS most commonly occurs in patients being treated with NRTIs, and is associated with hyperlactatemia or lactic acidosis, thought to caused by drug-induced mitochondrial toxicity. The pathologic mechanism underlying HANWS is incompletely understood. An acute axonal neuropathy is the most common finding, although demyelinating neuropathy and myopathy have also been reported. Treatment of HANWS is supportive and includes cessation of the NRTI and correction of metabolic abnormalities. Immunomodulatory therapies such as IVIg, and supplements including B vitamins, carnitine, and coenzyme Q have been used, but their efficacy is unclear.

Mononeuropathy multiplex

Mononeuropathy multiplex (MM), an uncommon complication of HIV infection, is defined as dysfunction of two or more peripheral nerves. As the individual nerves involved are variable, presenting complaints differ between patients. Common features include focal, asymmetric, sensory and motor deficits consistent with the distribution of one or more peripheral nerves. The incidence of MM has a bimodal distribution, with peaks in early and advanced HIV infection. In relatively immunocompetent patients, MM typically presents with dysfunction attributable to a limited number of cranial or peripheral nerves. The deficits typically resolve spontaneously over several months [33]. Although the initial presentation of MM in patients with advanced immunosuppression may be similar, the process rapidly spreads to involve multiple nerves, and the prognosis for recovery is much poorer [34].

The phenotypic dichotomy between early and late MM likely reflects differing pathogenic mechanisms. An autoimmune mechanism is postulated for early MM, whereas late MM may be related to CMV infection [35]. In both forms axonal degeneration and inflammation are seen in nerve biopsy specimens. This pattern is distinctive from MM in the general population, which is more often vasculitic.

NCS and EMG are the most helpful diagnostic studies in confirming the diagnosis of MM and assessing its severity. NCS reveals decreased motor and sensory evoked response amplitudes in specific nerves, with relative sparing of conduction velocities. Normal NCS in other nerves confirms the multifocality of the disorder and helps to distinguish it from polyneuropathy. EMG shows denervation in muscles supplied by affected nerves. Cerebrospinal fluid examination is helpful to document a positive CMV polymerase chain reaction in late MM; other changes are nonspecific. Nerve biopsy may be considered to rule out a vasculitic etiology.

Early MM does not necessarily require treatment; however, corticosteroids, IVIg, or plasmapheresis may hasten recovery. Numerous investigators recommend that late MM should be treated with empiric antiviral therapy, such as ganciclovir, foscarnet, and cidofovir, for presumed CMV infection, regardless of whether the organism can be demonstrated in cerebrospinal fluid, (preferably with PCR assay) or nerve biopsy.

Progressive polyradiculopathy

Like late MM, progressive polyradiculopathy is a rapidly progressive neurologic condition, usually associated with CMV infection in advanced AIDS patients [36]. Progressive polyradiculopathy results from CMV-induced inflammation and necrosis of lumbosacral roots at the level of the cauda equina. Lower extremity weakness and sphincter dysfunction develop, and neurologic examination reveals a flaccid paraparesis, hypore-flexia, and poor rectal tone. Upper extremities and cranial nerves are spared in all but the most severe cases.

Gadolinium enhanced MRI of the lumbosacral spine is mandatory to ex-clude compression of the cauda equina, but is either normal or demonstrates meningeal enhancement. A marked polymorphonuclear pleocytosis, with as many as 2,000 cells/mm^3, is the most dramatic cerebrospinal fluid abnormal-ity; low glucose, elevated protein, and a positive CMV PCR are also char-acteristic [37]. Neurophysiologic studies reveal diffusely decreased motor and sensory responses in the lower extremities, with prolonged or absent late responses and evidence of denervation on EMG. Long-term, empiric antiviral treatment, discussed above for late MM, is indicated for progres-sive polyradiculopathy; nevertheless, prognosis is poor and many patients do not improve.

Myopathy

Myopathy occurs as a complication of HIV, and also as a side effect of ARV treatment, in particular zidovudine (AZT). The presentation of HIV-associated myopathy is similar to other myopathies, with slowly pro-gressive, symmetric, predominantly proximal weakness [38]. Patients may report difficulty with tasks that stress proximal muscles, such as climbing stairs, rising from a low chair, or reaching for objects above the head. Mus-cular pain may not be present and is nonspecific. Less common presenta-tions include a wasting syndrome characterized by weight loss and generalized weakness, and an acute rhabdomyolysis with weakness, myalgia, and markedly elevated creatine kinase (CK) levels [39,40].

Neurologic examination reveals proximal weakness, including neck flex-ion, hip flexion, and shoulder abduction. Subtle weakness may be elicited by asking the patient to perform a deep knee bend or to keep the arms held aloft. Sensory examination is normal, and deep tendon reflexes are pre-served except in the setting of severe muscle wasting.

Diagnostic evaluation should include serum CK level, NCS, and EMG. NCS is most often normal, unless there is coexistent neuropathy. EMG re-veals brief, polyphasic motor units with early recruitment, most prominent in proximal muscles. Spontaneous activity may also be present. Muscle bi-opsy, if performed, may reveal myofiber degeneration, inflammatory infil-trate, inclusion bodies, and mitochondrial abnormalities [41].

The abnormalities seen on muscle biopsy have led to various proposed mechanisms for HIV-associated myopathy. The presence of inflammation suggests an immune-mediated etiology, which may primarily involve macro-phages and CD8+ T-cells [42]. Mitochondrial abnormalities have raised the issue of mitochondrial toxicity as an etiology, particularly in myopathy as-sociated with AZT [43].

If the patient is receiving AZT or other NRTI with mitochondrial toxicity, treatment begins with drug withdrawal if possible. Immunomodulatory therapies, such as IVIg or corticosteroids, may also be of use, although there are not controlled studies [44].

Other neuromuscular diseases

Herpes zoster is a reactivation of latent varicella zoster virus infection, which causes a painful, pruritic, vesicular rash in a dermatomal distribution. Herpes zoster occurs in HIV-negative patients as well, but the immunocompromised status of HIV-positive patients puts them at greater risk. The acute illness is commonly treated with antivirals and possibly corticosteroids. Postherpetic neuralgia, a syndrome of chronic pain in the same distribution as the rash, may subsequently develop. The management of postherpetic neuralgia is similar to that described for DSP.

Although there have been reports of other neuromuscular disorders in HIV-positive patients, such as myasthenia gravis and an Amyotrophic Lateral Sclerosis-like disease, a causal relationship has not been established [45,46]. Sensory neuronopathy, a primary sensory ataxia, has been described in several patients [47].

Summary

Neurologic complications of HIV infection are common, and are a significant source of morbidity. The chronic nature of HIV today, the complexity of highly active antiretroviral therapy regimens, and the multiple and diffuse effects of HIV on the nervous system present an exciting diagnostic challenge. A systematic, comprehensive approach to diagnosis and treatment is necessary, and can lead to substantial improvement in patients' quality of life.

References

[1] Morgello S, Estanislao L, Simpson D, et al. HIV-associated distal sensory polyneuropathy in the era of highly active antiretroviral therapy: the Manhattan HIV brain bank. Arch Neurol 2004;61:546–51.

[2] Simpson DM, Kitch D, Evans SR, et al. HIV neuropathy natural history cohort study: assessment measures and risk factors. Neurology 2006;66:1679–87.

[3] Pardo CA, McArthur JC, Griffin JW. HIV neuropathy: insights in the pathology of HIV peripheral nerve disease. J Peripher Nerv Syst 2001;6:21–7.

[4] Keswani SC, Polley M, Pardo CA, et al. Schwann cell chemokine receptors mediate HIV-1 gp120 toxicity to sensory neurons. Ann Neurol 2003;54:287–96.

[5] Simpson DM, Tagliati M. Nucleoside analogue-associated peripheral neuropathy in human immunodeficiency virus infection. J Acquir Immune Defic Syndr Hum Retrovirol 1995;9:153–61.

[6] Pettersen JA, Jones G, Worthington C, et al. Sensory neuropathy in human immunodeficiency virus/acquired immunodeficiency syndrome patients: protease inhibitor-mediated neurotoxicity. Ann Neurol 2006;59:816–24.

[7] Herrmann DN, McDermott MP, Sowden JE, et al. Is skin biopsy a predictor of transition to symptomatic HIV neuropathy? A longitudinal study. Neurology 2006;66:857–61.

[8] Berger AR, Arezzo JC, Schaumburg HH, et al. 2',3'-dideoxycytidine (ddC) toxic neuropathy: a study of 52 patients. Neurology 1993;43:358–62.

[9] Lesser H, Sharma U, LaMoreaux L, et al. Pregabalin relieves symptoms of painful diabetic neuropathy: a randomized controlled trial. Neurology 2004;63:2104–10.

[10] Rosenstock J, Tuchman M, LaMoreaux L, et al. Pregabalin for the treatment of painful diabetic peripheral neuropathy: a double-blind, placebo-controlled trial. Pain 2004;110:628–38.

[11] Hahn K, Arendt G, Braun JS, et al. A placebo-controlled trial of gabapentin for painful HIV-associated sensory neuropathies. J Neurol 2004;251:1260–6.

[12] Simpson DM, McArthur JC, Olney R, et al. Lamotrigine for HIV-associated painful sensory neuropathies: a placebo-controlled trial. Neurology 2003;60:1508–14.

[13] Atli A, Dogra S. Zonisamide in the treatment of painful diabetic neuropathy: a randomized, double-blind, placebo-controlled pilot study. Pain Med 2005;6:225–34.

[14] Raskin P, Donofrio PD, Rosenthal NR, et al. Topiramate vs placebo in painful diabetic neuropathy: analgesic and metabolic effects. Neurology 2004;63:865–73.

[15] Dogra S, Beydoun S, Mazzola J, et al. Oxcarbazepine in painful diabetic neuropathy: a randomized, placebo-controlled study. Eur J Pain 2005;9:543–54.

[16] Raskin J, Pritchett YL, Wang F, et al. A double-blind, randomized multicenter trial comparing duloxetine with placebo in the management of diabetic peripheral neuropathic pain. Pain Med 2005;6:346–56.

[17] Eli Lilly and Co. Cymbalta (duloxetine) product information. Available at: http://pi.lilly.com/us/cymbalta-pi.pdf. Accessed May, 2007.

[18] AstraZeneca. Elavil (amitiptyline) professional information brochure. Available at: http://www.fda.gov/cder/foi/label/2001/12704s45lbl.pdf.

[19] Estanislao L, Carter K, McArthur J, et al. Lidoderm-HIV Neuropathy Group. A randomized controlled trial of 5% lidocaine gel for HIV-associated distal symmetric polyneuropathy. J Acquir Immune Defic Syndr 2004;37:1584–6.

[20] Simpson D, Brown S, Tobias J. Treatment of painful HIV-associated distal sensory polyneuropathy (DSP) with a high-concentration capsaicin dermal patch (NGX-4010): report of a 52-week study. Program and Abstracts of the 59th Annual Meeting of the American Academy of Neurology. Boston, MA, April 28–May 5, 2007. Abstract S50.001.

[21] Portenoy RK, Bennett DS, Rauck R, et al. Prevalence and characteristics of breakthrough pain in opioid-treated patients with chronic noncancer pain. J Pain 2006;7:583–91.

[22] Cancer pain relief and palliative care. Report of a WHO expert committee. World Health Organ Tech Rep Ser 1990;804:1–75.

[23] Eisenberg E, McNicol ED, Carr DB. Efficacy and safety of opioid agonists in the treatment of neuropathic pain of nonmalignant origin: systematic review and meta-analysis of randomized controlled trials. JAMA 2005;293:3043–52.

[24] Simpson DM, Messina J, Xie F, et al. Fentanyl buccal tablet (FBT) for the treatment of breakthrough pain in opioid-tolerant patients with neuropathic pain: efficacy and patient preference outcomes from a double-blind, placebo-controlled study. 59th Annual Meeting of the American Academy of Neurology. Boston (MA), May 1, 2007.

[25] Rogstad KE, Shah R, Tesfaladet G, et al. Cardiovascular autonomic neuropathy in HIV infected patients. Sex Transm Infect 1999;75:264–7.

[26] Chimelli L, Martins AR. Degenerative and inflammatory lesions in sympathetic ganglia: further morphological evidence for an autonomic neuropathy in AIDS. J NeuroAIDS 2002;2:67–82.

[27] Cornblath DR, McArthur JC, Kennedy PG, et al. Inflammatory demyelinating peripheral neuropathies associated with human T-cell lymphotropic virus type III infection. Ann Neurol 1987;21:32–40.

[28] Morgello S, Simpson DM. Multifocal cytomegalovirus demyelinative polyneuropathy associated with AIDS. Muscle Nerve 1994;17:176–82.

[29] Arranz Caso JA, Martinez R, Cabrera F, et al. Miller fisher syndrome in a patient with HIV infection. AIDS 1997;11:550–1.

[30] Sillevis Smitt PA, Portegies P. Fisher's syndrome associated with human immunodeficiency virus infection. Clin Neurol Neurosurg 1990;92:353–5.

[31] Randomised trial of plasma exchange, intravenous immunoglobulin, and combined treatments in Guillain-Barre syndrome. Plasma exchange/sandoglobulin Guillain-Barre syndrome trial group. Lancet 1997;349:225–30.

[32] HIV Neuromuscular Syndrome Study Group. HIV-associated neuromuscular weakness syndrome. AIDS 2004;18:1403–12.

[33] Lipkin WI, Parry G, Kiprov D, et al. Inflammatory neuropathy in homosexual men with lymphadenopathy. Neurology 1985;35:1479–83.

[34] So Y, Olney R. The natural history of mononeuritis multiplex and simplex in HIV infection. Neurology 1991;41:375.

[35] Roullet E, Assuerus V, Gozlan J, et al. Cytomegalovirus multifocal neuropathy in AIDS: analysis of 15 consecutive cases. Neurology 1994;44:2174–82.

[36] Miller RG, Storey JR, Greco CM. Ganciclovir in the treatment of progressive AIDS-related polyradiculopathy. Neurology 1990;40:569–74.

[37] Kim YS, Hollander H. Polyradiculopathy due to cytomegalovirus: report of two cases in which improvement occurred after prolonged therapy and review of the literature. Clin Infect Dis 1993;17:32–7.

[38] Simpson DM, Bender AN. Human immunodeficiency virus-associated myopathy: analysis of 11 patients. Ann Neurol 1988;24:79–84.

[39] Simpson DM, Bender AN, Farraye J, et al. Human immunodeficiency virus wasting syndrome may represent a treatable myopathy. Neurology 1990;40:535–8.

[40] Chariot P, Ruet E, Authier FJ, et al. Acute rhabdomyolysis in patients infected by human immunodeficiency virus. Neurology 1994;44:1692–6.

[41] Simpson DM, Citak KA, Godfrey E, et al. Myopathies associated with human immunodeficiency virus and zidovudine: can their effects be distinguished? Neurology 1993;43:971–6.

[42] Illa I, Nath A, Dalakas M. Immunocytochemical and virological characteristics of HIV-associated inflammatory myopathies: similarities with seronegative polymyositis. Ann Neurol 1991;29:474–81.

[43] Dalakas MC, Illa I, Pezeshkpour GH, et al. Mitochondrial myopathy caused by long-term zidovudine therapy. N Engl J Med 1990;322:1098–105.

[44] Johnson RW, Williams FM, Kazi S, et al. Human immunodeficiency virus-associated polymyositis: a longitudinal study of outcome. Arthritis Rheum 2003;49:172–8.

[45] Nath A, Kerman RH, Novak IS, et al. Immune studies in human immunodeficiency virus infection with myasthenia gravis: a case report. Neurology 1990;40:581–3.

[46] Moulignier A, Moulonguet A, Pialoux G, et al. Reversible ALS-like disorder in HIV infection. Neurology 2001;57:995–1001.

[47] Elder G, Dalakas M, Pezeshkpour G, et al. Ataxic neuropathy due to ganglioneuronitis after probable acute human immunodeficiency virus infection. Lancet 1986;2:1275–6.

Phys Med Rehabil Clin N Am
19 (2008) 97–110

PHYSICAL MEDICINE
AND REHABILITATION
CLINICS OF
NORTH AMERICA

Critical Illness Neuromyopathy

Brent P. Goodman, MD[a,b,*], Andrea J. Boon, MD[c,d]

[a]*Department of Neurology, Mayo College of Medicine, Mayo Clinic,*
13400 East Shea Boulevard, Scottsdale, AZ 85259, USA
[b]*Electromyogram Laboratory, Mayo Clinic, 13400 East Shea Boulevard,*
Scottsdale, AZ 85259, USA
[c]*Department of Physical Medicine and Rehabilitation, Mayo College of Medicine,*
Mayo Clinic, 200 1st Street SW, Rochester, MN 55905, USA
[d]*Department of Neurology, Mayo College of Medicine, Mayo Clinic, 200 1st Street SW,*
Rochester, MN 55905, USA

Severe, generalized weakness is an increasingly recognized complication in patients who have critical illness. Before the advent of modern cardiopulmonary support in the intensive care unit (ICU), high mortality rates precluded clinical recognition of neuromuscular disorders associated with critical illness. In that era, the primary neuromuscular disorders recognized in critically ill patients were those such as myasthenia gravis and Guillain-Barre syndrome, which typically preceded, and occasionally resulted in, sepsis or multiple organ failure. As medical and surgical improvements led to improved survival of patients who have critical illness, a distinct neuromuscular syndrome was recognized and reported [1]. Electrodiagnostic studies revealed a length-dependent, sensorimotor polyneuropathy, and eventually this condition was named critical illness polyneuropathy [2].

Early electrophysiologic and morphologic studies in patients who had critical illness polyneuropathy also showed abnormalities of muscle fibers [3], and myopathy associated with critical illness was later recognized in many forms [4–7]. Ultimately an all-encompassing term, critical illness myopathy [8], was proposed. Although the relative frequency of critical illness myopathy and polyneuropathy remains the source of some controversy, it is now recognized that many, if not most, patients have electrophysiologic and morphologic evidence of both [9]. Despite reviews that consider the topic of critical illness polyneuropathy and myopathy separately (including this one), it may be more useful for the practicing clinician to approach the weak,

---

* Corresponding author. Department of Neurology, Mayo College of Medicine, Mayo Clinic, 13400 East Shea Boulevard, Scottsdale, AZ 85259.
E-mail address: goodman.brent@mayo.edu (B.P. Goodman).

critically ill patient as having a possible critical illness neuromyopathy. Such an approach reminds the evaluating clinician to be alert for features of both myopathy and polyneuropathy, which has important implications in terms of prognosis [9], and for future research studies focusing on pathogenesis and treatment of these disorders.

Approach to the critically ill patient who has limb and respiratory muscle weakness

Neuromuscular manifestations of critical illness are typically first recognized as failure to successfully wean from mechanical ventilation, or as generalized limb weakness. Careful review of past medical history and previous medical records, including collateral history from family and acquaintances, is important to establish the presence of a neurological condition that preceded the development of critical illness. Neuromuscular conditions, such as motor neuron disease, myasthenia gravis, Lambert-Eaton myasthenic syndrome, or Gullain-Barre syndrome, can lead to respiratory failure and pneumonia caused by aspiration, particularly when the respiratory and bulbar muscles are involved. Rapidly progressive acute and subacute infectious or neoplastic disorders, causing myelopathy or polyradiculopathy, need to be considered. Occasionally these disorders elude diagnosis, or progress so rapidly that diagnosis is not possible before admission to the ICU.

A systematic, localization-based approach, considering possible involvement of the brain, spinal cord, peripheral nerves, muscle, or neuromuscular junction is important (Box 1). Septic encephalopathy is an early and very common manifestation of critical illness, occurring in as many as 70% of patients who have critical illness [1,10,11]. Encephalopathy in critical illness reflects functional, not structural, disease [12]. The presence of focal signs on examination, such as hemiparesis, asymmetric hyperreflexia, or Babinski signs, should prompt further diagnostic testing, such as head CT or brain MRI, and cerebrospinal fluid testing. Spinal cord imaging with either CT or MRI should also be considered for critically ill patients who have weakness and upper motor neuron signs, such as hyperreflexia and Babinski signs, on examination.

Electrodiagnostic testing, including nerve conduction studies (NCS), needle electromyography (EMG), and repetitive nerve stimulation (RNS), provides the best opportunity to characterize the cause of weakness as a disorder of anterior horn cells, peripheral nerve, muscle, or neuromuscular junction. RNS is used to determine the presence of a neuromuscular junction disorder such as myasthenia gravis, Lambert-Eaton myasthenic syndrome, botulism, or transient neuromuscular blockade following administration of a neuromuscular blocking agent. Serum creatine kinase (CK) determination and muscle biopsy is occasionally used to characterize the nature of a suspected myopathy.

Box 1. Differential diagnosis of weakness in the intensive care unit

Muscle disorders
Acid maltase disease
Dystrophinopathies
Critical illness myopathy
Polymyositis/dermatomyositis

Neuromuscular junction disorders
Myasthenia gravis
Lambert-Eaton myasthenic syndrome
Botulism
Neuromuscular blocking agents

Neuropathy/motor neuron disorders
Guillian-Barre syndrome
Chronic inflammatory demyelinating polyradiculoneuropathy
Motor neuron disease
West Nile encephalomyelitis

Spinal cord disorders
Ischemia
Hemorrhage
Trauma
Neoplasm

Sepsis, multiple organ failure, and systemic inflammatory response syndrome

Critical illness refers to the syndrome of sepsis and multiple organ failure. Sepsis has historically been defined as a severe, systemic response to infection. The concept of the systemic inflammatory response syndrome (SIRS) was developed to clarify terminology, acknowledging that a severe systemic inflammatory response occurs in noninfectious disorders such as trauma [9]. Sepsis is applied in the SIRS when infection has been documented.

Clinical manifestations of SIRS have been established, including: (1) body temperature of greater than 38°C or les than36°C; (2) heart rate greater than 90; (3) tachypnea, indicated by respiratory rate greater than 20 or $PaCo_2$ of less than 32; (4) abnormal white blood cell count, either greater than 12,000 cells/mm^3 or less than 4000 cells/mm^3, or less than 10% "bands" (Fig. 1) [13].

Humoral and cellular responses are activated in SIRS and sepsis, which produce diffuse microcirculatory changes throughout the body [14]. The humoral response is triggered by epithelial cells, endothelial cells, macrophages

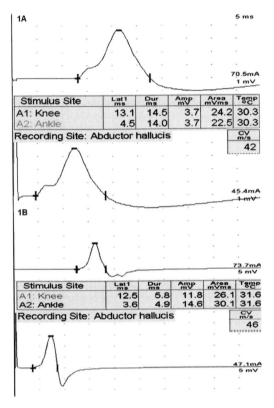

Fig. 1. Demonstration of prolonged CMAP duration in critical illness myopathy. Tibial motor nerve conduction study in a patient with critical illness myopathy (*1A*) compared with normal control (*1B*). Sweep speed 5 ms/division in both studies. The compound muscle action potential duration in 1A is over twice the duration in 1 B, but there is no decomposition of the wave form or dispersion between proximal and distal sites of stimulation.

and neutrophils, which induce proinflammatory cytokines such as interleukins-1, -2, and -6, tumor necrosis factor (TNF)-α and free radicals [9]. Adhesion molecules adhere to endothelial cells, platelets, and leukocytes, which leads to capillary obstruction and subsequent endothelial damage [9]. Endothelial damage results in tissue edema and promotes a prothrombotic state [9,15]. The cumulative impact of these changes results in microcirculatory disturbances, which impair energy substrate delivery to end organs, thereby causing organ dysfunction or failure [16].

Critical illness polyneuropathy develops in 50% to 70% of patients who have sepsis [1]. At least 33% of ICU patients treated for status asthmaticus develop critical illness myopathy [7], and in patients undergoing liver transplantation, critical illness myopathy develops in 7% [17]. The prevalence of critical illness myopathy in SIRS is unknown.

Critical illness polyneuropathy

Patients who have critical illness polyneuropathy develop distal weakness, may have depressed deep tendon reflexes, and not uncommonly fail to wean from mechanical ventilation. Sensory loss may be difficult to demonstrate, given the high prevalence of encephalopathy in critical illness; however, in a patient with spontaneous limb movements, failure to withdraw a limb following administration of painful stimulation to the distal limb suggests sensory loss. Cranial nerve abnormalities are exceedingly rare and should suggest an alternative diagnosis.

Electrodiagnostic features

Thoughtful electrodiagnostic testing is important in the evaluation of suspected critical illness polyneuropathy. Upper and lower limb motor and sensory NCS are performed. In patients who have suspected respiratory muscle failure, phrenic NCS are also performed. RNS is normal in critical illness polyneuropathy, and is helpful to exclude a pre-existing neuromuscular junction disorder or weakness caused by transient neuromuscular blockade following administration of a neuromuscular junction blocking agent. Because the majority of patients are too weak to exercise, brief, high-frequency repetitive stimulation (at 20 or 50 Hz x 1–2 seconds) should be performed to evaluate for significant facilitation of the compound muscle action potential amplitude. This is particularly important if low-amplitude compound muscle action potentials (CMAP) are present with routine NCS, typically seen in the Lambert-Eaton myasthenic syndrome. Motor CMAP amplitudes and sensory nerve action potential (SNAP) amplitudes are typically reduced, with normal or near normal conduction velocities and distal latencies. Decline in the CMAP amplitudes occurs early in the course of the illness, and may be followed by subsequent decline in the SNAP amplitudes later [9,18]. Significant conduction velocity slowing or distal latency prolongation and features of temporal dispersion or conduction block should suggest an alternative diagnosis, such as Guillain-Barre syndrome.

Needle EMG typically shows abnormal spontaneous activity in distal muscles, and may show reduced recruitment of motor unit potentials. The presence of small motor unit potentials on needle EMG should alert the electromyographer to the possibility of a concomitant myopathy, particularly if the SNAP amplitudes are normal or near-normal. Single-fiber EMG studies in nine patients who had critical illness polyneuropathy showed increased jitter, suggesting a disorder of nerve terminals in these patients [19]; however, assessment of motor unit potentials can be difficult in the encephalopathic patient, who may be unable to activate motor unit potentials. In a patient who has low-amplitude CMAPs and preserved SNAPs, and who is unable to activate motor unit potentials, it may not be possible with routine electrodiagnostic studies to determine whether the patient has a myopathy, polyneuropathy, or both. Prolonged CMAP duration and muscle inexcitability on direct muscle stimulation suggests the presence of myopathy. In such a patient, repeat NCS and needle EMG should be considered following improvement in encephalopathy or weakness.

Pathology and pathophysiology

Nerve biopsy and postmortem autopsy studies showed evidence of primary axonal degeneration, without findings of inflammation or primary demyelination [2,20]. Axonal degeneration of intercostal and phrenic nerves and denervation atrophy in respiratory muscles was felt to explain the respiratory insufficiency in these patients [2].

The cause of critical illness polyneuropathy is speculative. Many different factors have been hypothesized in the pathogenesis of critical illness polyneuropathy. No drug, toxin, infection, nutritional deficiency, or iatrogenic agent has been identified as being causative. It is likely that systemic physiologic changes associated with sepsis, multiple organ failure, and the SIRS cause critical illness polyneuropathy. Critical illness neuropathy severity has been associated with ICU length of stay, elevated serum glucose levels, and decreased serum albumin levels [10]. Critically ill patients who have high APACHE (Acute Physiology, Age, Chronic Health Evaluation)-III score and the SIRS are most prone to the development of critical illness neuropathy [21].

The current, prevailing hypothesis is that cytokines secreted in sepsis increase microvascular permeability [2], resulting in endoneural edema, leading to failure of distal axonal transport and subsequent axonal degeneration [9]. The lack of peripheral nerve microvascular autoregulation likely enhances susceptibility to such a process [14]. The role of a neurotoxin in critical illness neuropathy has been suggested [22] but not definitively demonstrated.

Critical illness myopathy

The predominant clinical feature of critical illness myopathy is that of a diffuse, flaccid weakness, typically involving limb, neck, diaphragm, and even facial muscles. Deep tendon reflexes may be decreased, and if elicitable, the sensory examination may be normal. The presence of critical illness myopathy is typically suspected following recovery from sedation and encephalopathy, and patients frequently exhibit difficulty weaning from mechanical ventilation. Diagnostic features have been proposed for critical illness myopathy (Box 2). These features are best reserved for research protocols.

Electrodiagnostic features

NCS in patients who have critical illness myopathy typically show low amplitude CMAPs, with preserved conduction velocities and distal latencies. The authors and others have observed prolongation of CMAP duration to be a specific feature of critical illness myopathy (see Fig. 1) [2,23,24].

Box 2. Proposed diagnostic features for critical illness myopathy

Major diagnostic features
1. SNAP amplitudes greater than 80% lower limit of normal for two or more nerves
2. Small motor unit potentials (MUPs) on needle EMG, with or without fibrillation potentials
3. Absence of decrement on RNS
4. Myosin loss on muscle biopsy

Supportive diagnostic features
1. CMAP amplitudes less than 80% lower limit of normal in two or more nerves without conduction block
2. Elevated serum CK
3. Demonstration of muscle inexcitability

For a definite diagnosis of critical illness myopathy, patients should have all four major diagnostic features. For probable critical illness myopathy, patients should have three major, and at least one supportive diagnostic feature. For possible critical illness myopathy, patients should have major features 1 and 3, or 2 and 3, and at least one supportive diagnostic feature

---

From Lacomis D, Zochodne DW, Bird SJ. Critical illness myopathy. Muscle Nerve 2000;23(12):1787; with permission. Copyright © 2000, Wiley Periodicals, Inc., A Wiley Company.

CMAP duration may be normal or only mildly prolonged if NCS are performed early in the patient's illness, but appear to become more prolonged later in the patient's course, and subsequently shorten with recovery. SNAP amplitudes are typically preserved; however, low SNAP amplitudes can be seen in patients who have concomitant critical illness polyneuropathy or preexisting disease such as diabetic neuropathy, or can be decreased because of technical factors such as limb edema. RNS studies are normal in critical illness myopathy.

Needle EMG in critical illness myopathy frequently shows abnormal spontaneous activity, including fibrillation potentials and positive sharp waves. With voluntary activation, rapid recruitment of small motor unit potentials is typical. As discussed previously, some patients, because of encephalopathy, sedation, or profound muscle weakness, are unable to voluntarily activate motor unit potentials. In these patients, determining whether a patient has critical illness myopathy or neuropathy can be difficult. In such patients, the presence of reduced CMAP amplitudes, prolonged CMAP durations, and preserved SNAPs are most suggestive of critical illness myopathy.

The technique of direct muscle stimulation can be of benefit in distinguishing critical illness polyneuropathy from critical illness myopathy.

Using this technique, it has been demonstrated that muscle in critical illness myopathy is electrically inexcitable, whereas in critical illness polyneuropathy a large potential can be elicited with direct muscle stimulation [25,26]. This is hypothesized to result from abnormal sodium channel inactivation in critical illness myopathy [27]. Similar pathophysiology likely explains the finding of CMAP duration in critical illness myopathy.

Pathology and pathophysiology

Muscle biopsy findings can be quite variable in patients who have critical illness myopathy. Atrophy of type 1 fibers only, type 2 fibers, or of all fiber types has been reported [5]. Thick filament myosin loss seen on light and electron microscopy has been the most frequently reported pathological finding [5,6,28,29], and has historically been associated with the term acute quadriplegic myopathy (Fig. 2). Necrosis is not a common morphologic feature, though widespread necrosis has been reported in some patients, with so-called "acute necrotizing myopathy of intensive care" [4,30]. These patients generally have severe quadriparesis, marked serum CK elevation, and myoglobinuria.

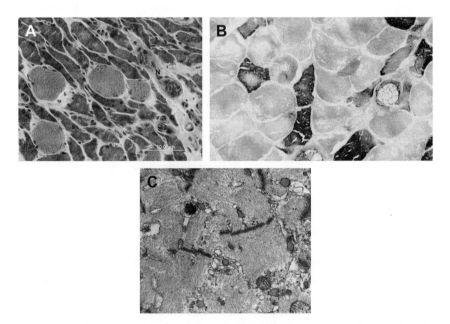

Fig. 2. (*A*) Trichrome stained section showing many small fibers among few of normal size. The small fibers have different staining properties and contain fine granular material. (*B*) Myosin AT-Pase (pH4.3) reacted section in which type 1 fibers should stain dark and the other fibers more faintly. Several reactive fibers show irregularly circumscribed decreases of reactivity and all remaining fibers fail to react. (*C*) Electron micrograph showing disarrayed myofibrils devoid of thick filaments that consist only of thin filaments emanating from Z disks (Z). Dislocated sarcotubular profiles and mitochondria are scattered in the field. (*Courtesy of* AG Engel, MD, Rochester, MN.)

High dose corticosteroids, non-depolarizing neuromuscular blocking agents, and sedating agents such as propofol [31] are putative risk factors for the development of critical illness myopathy; however, sepsis and the systemic inflammatory response syndrome seem to be the most significant risk factors. Critical illness myopathy has been reported to occur in patients who have not been exposed to corticosteroids or neuromuscular junction blocking agents [25,32,33]. Some authors have proposed that these risk factors contribute to muscle inactivity [27], which may be important in the pathogenesis of critical illness myopathy.

In an animal model of critical illness myopathy, muscle denervation followed by corticosteroid administration results in a myosin-loss myopathy [34,35]. Prolonged neuromuscular junction blockade by neuromuscular blocking agents has been hypothesized to cause muscle denervation [36]. In this model, the cumulative effects of disturbed microcirculation, in conjunction with neuromuscular blocking agents, result in muscle denervation, which in turn can result in myopathy following corticosteroid administration.

More recent studies suggest disordered muscle membrane properties in critical illness myopathy, congruent with electrodiagnostic findings showing increased CMAP duration and loss of muscle excitability with direct muscle stimulation. In animal models, denervated muscle fibers that are exposed to corticosteroids become electrically inexcitable [37]. In this model, several different electrophysiologic changes contribute to inexcitability, including depolarization of the resting membrane potential, loss of sodium channels on muscle membrane, and change in voltage-dependent inactivation of sodium channels [37,38].

Although functional changes in muscle membrane excitability appear to play a major role in the pathogenesis of critical illness myopathy, structural changes such as myosin loss are also prominent. In one study [39], a decrease in myosin RNA correlated with reduced myosin levels in muscle, suggesting that altered gene expression likely plays an important role. Altered calcium homeostasis may be important in the development of myosin deficiency. The expression of calpain, a calcium-activated protease, was found to be increased in atrophic muscle fibers [5]. This proteolytic cascade is involved in the breakdown of myosin and other muscle proteins such as titin, nebulin, and actin, all of which appear to be reduced in critical illness myopathy [27]. A comprehensive understanding of critical illness myopathy pathogenesis must account for features of altered gene expression, disordered muscle membrane function, and proteolytic pathways involved in muscle protein breakdown.

Combined critical illness polyneuropathy and myopathy: critical illness neuromyopathy

Early studies by Bolton and colleagues reported myopathic features, including cytoarchitectural disorganization and necrosis, in addition to chronic denervation [2,20]. Another early study by Op de Coul and colleagues [40] reported concomitant involvement of nerve and muscle in ICU patients exposed to a neuromuscular blocking agent; however, as later studies attempted to define the fundamental electrophysiologic and pathologic findings in the polyneuropathy and myopathy of critical illness, there appeared to be a waning appreciation or acceptance of coexistent polyneuropathy and myopathy in these patients. Furthermore, there has been controversy in the literature in regard to the relative frequency of critical illness polyneuropathy and myopathy. In a prospective 1996 study of 24 quadriplegic, critically ill patients, muscle biopsy revealed evidence of myopathy in 23, whereas only 8 had abnormalities on nerve biopsy [41]. The relative infrequency of sural nerve biopsy abnormalities in this study was somewhat surprising, given that NCS showed evidence of polyneuropathy in nearly all patients. A more recent prospective study reported NCS findings of polyneuropathy in 22 patients, with evidence of myopathy in all 10 patients in this series who underwent muscle biopsy [42].

These studies suggest that most critically ill patients who develop weakness have features of both polyneuropathy and myopathy on electrodiagnostic testing and muscle biopsy. It has been suggested that the predominance of neurogenic or myopathic features may depend upon the use of neuromuscular blocking agents and steroids [9]. In critically ill patients not exposed to these drugs, critical illness polyneuropathy may be the predominant manifestation [18], and in patients exposed to these drugs, critical illness myopathy may predominate [43].

Treatment and prognosis of critical illness polyneuropathy and myopathy

The primary, initial treatment approach involves the prevention and management of sepsis, SIRS, and multiple organ dysfunction. Because corticosteroids and neuromuscular blocking agents are important in pathogenesis, these agents should be avoided if at all possible. Aggressive treatment of infection, hypotension, and hypoxemia is paramount. Early and ongoing treatment of organ failure is important. Treatment approaches targeting the immunologic response to sepsis have largely been unsuccessful in preventing or improving the neuromuscular complications of critical illness.

Involvement of the physiatrist and associated team members is ideally initiated immediately following the recognition of neuromuscular disease in the ICU. Initially, stretching and passive range-of-motion exercises to maintain joint mobility and prevent contractures are begun. Respiratory therapy is important to minimize the risk of superimposed pulmonary infection. Skin protection measures should be initiated, with an appropriate mattress to optimize pressure relief and frequent turning of the patient to prevent the development of pressure ulcers. As the patient improves, therapy can be advanced, with gradual mobilization, progressive strengthening of the major upper and lower extremity muscle groups, and training in activities of daily living. It is important that progressive resistance training is submaximal, to prevent excessive fatigue of the recovering nerve terminals and muscle fibers.

Most patients will benefit from transitioning to an inpatient rehabilitation unit once clinically stable, with the goal of returning home to independent living. Disposition at discharge will be influenced by the functional deficits at the time of admission to the acute rehabilitation unit, the underlying pathophysiology of the disease process and associated rate of recovery, and the degree of social support available at home. A multidisciplinary approach, with continued involvement of the physical and occupational therapists, speech therapy if there is significant facial weakness that could contribute to dysarthria or dysphagia, and other team members such as a neuropsychologist and recreational therapist is optimal to maximize the patient's chance of returning to the premorbid level of function as quickly as possible. Many patients will initially need to function from a wheelchair base, and may require assistive devices and adapative equipment at the time of discharge home from the rehabilitation unit.

Long-term prognostic studies in patients who have critical illness myopathy and polyneuropathy are limited. In one study of 13 patients who had critical illness polyneuropathy, clinical and electrodiagnostic testing was performed at a mean of 17 months [44]. Only 2 of these patients had normal neurological examinations, NCS abnormalities were seen in all patients, and low quality of life scores were reported in the majority of patients. In a prospective study of long-term survivors of critical illness polyneuropathy/myopathy who underwent clinical and electrodiagnostic evaluation at a median time of 42.5 months following ICU discharge, persistent muscular weakness and needle EMG abnormalities were reported in 31% and 95% of survivors, respectively [45]. In another study of 19 patients who had critical illness polyneuropathy, 4 patients died between 2 and 9 months following diagnosis, 4 patients had significant, persistent weakness, including 2 who had complete quadriplegia, and complete recovery was reported in 8 patients [46].

Prognosis likely correlates with the severity of weakness and the degree of axonal degeneration. Patients who have severe critical illness polyneuropathy may remain quadriplegic [10]. In patients who have a predominantly myopathic process, absence of necrosis on muscle biopsy, and lack of serum CK elevation, a favorable outcome is likely even in cases with profound weakness [9]. Patients who have high serum CK elevations and necrosis on muscle biopsy have a less favorable prognosis [47].

Summary

Critical illness polyneuropathy and myopathy are frequent complications in critically ill patients who have sepsis or SIRS. Patients are typically diagnosed with these disorders when patients fail to wean off of ventilatory support (despite adequate cardiopulmonary status), or when severe limb weakness is noted during or following recovery from critical illness.

Exploration of past medical history to exclude pre-existing neuromuscular conditions and electrodiagnostic testing establishes the diagnosis.

NCS in both critical illness polyneuropathy and myopathy show low amplitude CMAPs, whereas reduction in SNAP amplitudes would be expected only in critical illness polyneuropathy. Needle EMG in both conditions can show abnormal spontaneous activity; however, in critical illness polyneuropathy, large motor unit potentials with reduced recruitment may be seen. Needle EMG in critical illness myopathy shows small motor unit potentials with rapid recruitment. In patients who are unable to voluntarily activate motor unit potentials, determining whether a polyneuropathy or myopathy is present can be difficult. The presence of prolonged CMAP durations and inexcitability on direct muscle stimulation suggest critical illness myopathy. It is now recognized that many patients who have critical illness can have both polyneuropathy and myopathy, so-called "critical illness neuromyopathy."

Pathogenesis of critical illness polyneuropathy and myopathy remains speculative, with corticosteroids and neuromuscular blocking agents recognized as the most significant risk factors. Treatment consists of avoidance of these agents, and is otherwise supportive. Future therapeutic interventions will require better understanding of disease pathogenesis, but may target pro-inflammatory cytokine and free-radical pathways, muscle gene expression, ion channel function, or proteolytic muscle protein mechanisms.

Rehabilitation is targeted initially toward maintenance of range of motion and prevention of contractures, with progression to gradual mobilization and submaximal strengthening as clinically indicated, and provision of adaptive equipment, to maximize functional independence. The literature on prognosis is limited, but in general, recovery is prolonged and often incomplete, particularly in patients who have severe quadriplegic myopathy who have elevated serum CK and necrosis on muscle biopsy.

References

[1] Bolton CF, Young GB, Zochodne DW. The neurological complications of sepsis. Ann Neurol 1993;33(1):94–100.
[2] Zochodne DW, Bolton CF, Wells GA, et al. Critical illness polyneuropathy. A complication of sepsis and multiple organ failure. Brain 1987;110(Pt 4):819–41.
[3] Zochodne DW, Bolton CF, Thompson RT, et al. Myopathy in critical illness. Muscle Nerve 1986;9:652.
[4] Zochodne DW, Ramsay DA, Saly V, et al. Acute necrotizing myopathy of intensive care: electrophysiological studies. Muscle Nerve 1994;17(3):285–92.
[5] Showalter CJ, Engel AG. Acute quadriplegic myopathy: analysis of myosin isoforms and evidence for calpain-mediated proteolysis. Muscle Nerve 1997;20(3):316–22.
[6] Lacomis D, Giuliani MJ, Van Cott A, et al. Acute myopathy of intensive care: clinical, electromyographic, and pathological aspects. Ann Neurol 1996;40(4):645–54.
[7] Douglass JA, Tuxen DV, Horne M, et al. Myopathy in severe asthma. Am Rev Respir Dis 1992;146(2):517–9.

[8] Lacomis D, Zochodne DW, Bird SJ. Critical illness myopathy. Muscle Nerve 2000;23(12): 1785–8.

[9] Bolton CF. Neuromuscular manifestations of critical illness. Muscle Nerve 2005;32(2): 140–63.

[10] Witt NJ, Zochodne DW, Bolton CF, et al. Peripheral nerve function in sepsis and multiple organ failure. Chest 1991;99(1):176–84.

[11] Young GB, Bolton CF, Austin TW, et al. The encephalopathy associated with septic illness. Clin Invest Med 1990;13(6):297–304.

[12] Jackson AC, Gilbert JJ, Young GB, et al. The encephalopathy of sepsis. Can J Neurol Sci 1985;12(4):303–7.

[13] Bone RC. Sepsis syndrome. New insights into its pathogenesis and treatment. Intensive Care World 1992;4:50–9.

[14] Bolton CF. Sepsis and the systemic inflammatory response syndrome: neuromuscular manifestations. Crit Care Med 1996;24(8):1408–16.

[15] Faust SN, Levin M, Harrison OB, et al. Dysfunction of endothelial protein C activation in severe meningococcal sepsis. N Engl J Med 2001;345(6):408–16.

[16] Glauser MP, Zanetti G, Baumgartner JD, et al. Septic shock: pathogenesis [see comment]. Lancet 1991;338(8769):732–6.

[17] Campellone JV, Lacomis D, Kramer DJ, et al. Acute myopathy after liver transplantation [see comment]. Neurology 1998;50(1):46–53.

[18] Zifko UA, Zipko HT, Bolton CF. Clinical and electrophysiological findings in critical illness polyneuropathy. J Neurol Sci 1998;159(2):186–93.

[19] Schwarz J, Planck J, Briegel J, et al. Single-fiber electromyography, nerve conduction studies, and conventional electromyography in patients with critical-illness polyneuropathy: evidence for a lesion of terminal motor axons. Muscle Nerve 1997;20(6):696–701.

[20] Bolton CF, Gilbert JJ, Hahn AF, et al. Polyneuropathy in critically ill patients. J Neurol Neurosurg Psychiatr 1984;47(11):1223–31.

[21] de Letter MA, Schmitz PI, Visser LH, et al. Risk factors for the development of polyneuropathy and myopathy in critically ill patients. Crit Care Med 2001;29(12):2281–6.

[22] Druschky A, Herkert M, Radespiel-Troger M, et al. Critical illness polyneuropathy: clinical findings and cell culture assay of neurotoxicity assessed by a prospective study. Intensive Care Med 2001;27(4):686–93.

[23] Park EJ, Nishida T, Sufit RL, et al. Prolonged compound muscle action potential duration in critical illness myopathy: report of nine cases. Clinical Neuromuscular Disease 2004;5: 176–83.

[24] Sandrock AW, Cros DP, Louis DN. Case 11: a 51-year-old man with chronic obstructive pulmonary disease and generalized muscle weakness. N Engl J Med 1997;336:1079–88.

[25] Rich MM, Bird SJ, Raps EC, et al. Direct muscle stimulation in acute quadriplegic myopathy. Muscle Nerve 1997;20(6):665–73.

[26] Trojaborg W, Weimer LH, Hays AP. Electrophysiologic studies in critical illness associated weakness: myopathy or neuropathy—a reappraisal. Clin Neurophysiol 2001;112(9): 1586–93.

[27] Bird SJ, Rich MM. Critical illness myopathy and polyneuropathy. Curr Neurol Neurosci Rep 2002;2(6):527–33.

[28] Faragher MW, Day BJ, Dennett X. Critical care myopathy: an electrophysiological and histological study. Muscle Nerve 1996;19(4):516–8.

[29] Sander HW, Golden M, Danon MJ. Quadriplegic areflexic ICU illness: selective thick filament loss and normal nerve histology. Muscle Nerve 2002;26(4):499–505.

[30] Coakley JH, Nagendran K, Honavar M, et al. Preliminary observations on the neuromuscular abnormalities in patients with organ failure and sepsis [see comment]. Intensive Care Med 1993;19(6):323–8.

[31] Hanson P, Dive A, Brucher JM, et al. Acute corticosteroid myopathy in intensive care patients. Muscle Nerve 1997;20(11):1371–80.

[32] Hirano M, Ott BR, Raps EC, et al. Acute quadriplegic myopathy: a complication of treatment with steroids, nondepolarizing blocking agents, or both [see comment]. Neurology 1992;42(11):2082–7.

[33] Hoke A, Rewcastle NB, Zochodne DW. Acute quadriplegic myopathy unrelated to steroids or paralyzing agents: quantitative EMG studies. Can J Neurol Sci 1999;26(4):325–9.

[34] Massa R, Carpenter S, Holland P, et al. Loss and renewal of thick myofilaments in glucocorticoid-treated rat soleus after denervation and reinnervation. Muscle Nerve 1992;15(11): 1290–8.

[35] Rouleau G, Karpati G, Carpenter S, et al. Glucocorticoid excess induces preferential depletion of myosin in denervated skeletal muscle fibers. Muscle Nerve 1987;10(5):428–38.

[36] Wernig A, Pecot-Dechavassine M, Stover H. Sprouting and regression of the nerve at the frog neuromuscular junction in normal conditions and after prolonged paralysis with curare. J Neurocytol 1980;9(3):278–303.

[37] Rich MM, Pinter MJ, Kraner SD, et al. Loss of electrical excitability in an animal model of acute quadriplegic myopathy [see comment]. Ann Neurol 1998;43(2):171–9.

[38] Rich MM, Pinter MJ. Sodium channel inactivation in an animal model of acute quadriplegic myopathy. Ann Neurol 2001;50(1):26–33.

[39] Larsson L, Li X, Edstrom L, et al. Acute quadriplegia and loss of muscle myosin in patients treated with nondepolarizing neuromuscular blocking agents and corticosteroids: mechanisms at the cellular and molecular levels. Crit Care Med 2000;28(1):34–45.

[40] Op de Coul AA, Verheul GA, Leyten AC, et al. Critical illness polyneuromyopathy after artificial respiration. Clin Neurol Neurosurg 1991;93(1):27–33.

[41] Latronico N, Fenzi F, Recupero D, et al. Critical illness myopathy and neuropathy. Lancet 1996;347(9015):1579–82.

[42] De Jonghe B, Sharshar T, Lefaucheur JP, et al. Paresis acquired in the intensive care unit: a prospective multicenter study. JAMA 2002;288(22):2859–67.

[43] Lacomis D, Petrella JT, Giuliani MJ. Causes of neuromuscular weakness in the intensive care unit: a study of ninety-two patients. Muscle Nerve 1998;21(5):610–7.

[44] Zifko UA. Long-term outcome of critical illness polyneuropathy. Muscle Nerve Suppl 2000; 9:S49–52.

[45] Fletcher SN, Kennedy DD, Ghosh IR, et al. Persistent neuromuscular and neurophysiologic abnormalities in long-term survivors of prolonged critical illness [see comment]. Crit Care Med 2003;31(4):1012–6.

[46] de Seze M, Petit H, Wiart L, et al. Critical illness polyneuropathy. A 2-year follow-up study in 19 severe cases. Eur Neurol 2000;43(2):61–9.

[47] Bolton CF, Ramsay DA, Rutledge F. Acute quadriplegic myopathy (AQM), spesis and the systemic inflammatory response syndrome (SIRS). Neurology 1998;50:242–3.

ELSEVIER
SAUNDERS

Phys Med Rehabil Clin N Am
19 (2008) 111–124

PHYSICAL MEDICINE
AND REHABILITATION
CLINICS OF
NORTH AMERICA

Neuromuscular Complications
of Bariatric Surgery

Pariwat Thaisetthawatkul, MD

Department of Neurological Sciences, University of Nebraska Medical Center,
982045 Nebraska Medical Center, Omaha, NE 68198–2045, USA

Obesity is defined as a body mass index (BMI) of greater than or equal to 30 kg/m^2. Severe obesity is defined as 100 lb above ideal body weight or as a BMI above 35 kg/m^2 [1]. Obesity has been shown to be associated with many comorbidities, such as cardiovascular-related disease, stroke, obstructive sleep apnea, type 2 diabetes mellitus, dyslipidemia, hypertension, hepatobiliary disease, cancer, endocrine disorders, psychosocial problems, and many orthopedic complications [2]. Management options for severe obesity can be divided into nonsurgical or surgical approaches. The nonsurgical approach includes behavioral treatment [3], nutritional modification [4], and drug treatment [5]. In the case of morbid obesity, however, conservative management has been disappointing [1]. In 1991, the National Institutes of Health issued a statement from a consensus conference panel recommending that surgical options or bariatric surgery be strongly considered in selected patients who have morbid obesity [6]. This type of surgery was developed around the 1950s as a result of observations on the consequence of patients who had short bowel syndrome [7]. After that, the procedures have been performed increasingly and become more popularized. The number of the procedures performed increased from 20,000 in 1993 to more than 120,000 in 2003 [8]. Bariatric surgery is very effective in initiating and maintaining weight loss, and in reducing comorbidities [9]. The procedures have been adopted by people from all walks of life. Generally, indications to consider bariatric surgery include 1) adult patients who have a BMI greater than 40 kg/m^2 or 2) adult patients who have a BMI between 35 and 40 kg/m^2 and have comorbid conditions such as cardiovascular diseases, severe diabetes mellitus, or hypertension [6]. To understand the pathophysiology of neuromuscular complications after bariatric surgery, it would be very helpful to review first the techniques: surgical and metabolic

---

E-mail address: pthaiset@unmc.edu

1047-9651/08/$ - see front matter © 2008 Elsevier Inc. All rights reserved.
doi:10.1016/j.pmr.2007.10.008

complications of bariatric surgery. Then, neuromuscular complications after the surgery will be reviewed.

Techniques of bariatric surgery and surgical complications

Bariatric surgery may be divided into three main types: restrictive, malabsorptive, and combined procedures [10]. Vertical banded gastroplasty (VBG) and gastric banding (GB) are examples of restrictive procedures.

In VBG, a small proximal gastric pouch (usually less than 20 mL in size) will be created [11]. This pouch is drained through a small outlet (usually 10 to 12 mm in diameter) along the lesser curvature of the stomach [12]. In pure restrictive procedures, normal absorption of nutrients through the small intestines is left intact. The procedure produces early satiety, and weight loss is achieved through reduced calorie intake. Because of this, nutritional deficiencies very uncommonly occur, unless there are complications such as severe nausea and vomiting, which can occur in about 8% of patients [13], or marked changes in eating habits [12].

Biliopancreatic diversion (BPD) is an example of malabsorptive procedure. This procedure was developed and popularized in Europe [14]. The procedure creates fat malabsorption by rerouting bile from entering the usual route, at proximal small intestine, to a common limb created at the distal ileum [14]. In BPD, a proximal gastric pouch, the size of which is about 100 to 150 mL, is created along the lesser curvature of the stomach [15]. The distal ileum is divided at about 250 cm from the ileocecal valve, and the distal stump is lifted and anastomosed to the created stomach pouch as an alimentary limb [14] The proximal stump is anastomosed to the alimentary limb as a side-to-side entero-enterostomy at about 50 to 100 cm from the ileocecal valve, thus creating a common channel, where the food, bile, and digestive enzymes can be mixed. The length of this common limb depends on how severe malabsorption is required in each individual. To reduce the risk of developing proximal duodenal ulcers after the procedure, distal gastrectomy may be performed [14]. This procedure results in significant weight loss but has many adverse effects, such as diarrhea, gall stones, malodorous stool and gas, vitamin and mineral deficiencies, especially fat-soluble vitamins, protein–calorie malnutrition, and bacterial overgrowth. The patients who have this procedure will need to have a close and life-long follow-up and nutritional care [14].

The most commonly performed bariatric procedure in the United States is Roux-en-Y gastric bypass (RYGB) [8]. This combined procedure uses a small gastric pouch (10 to 30 mL), which is drained to 75 to 150 cm Roux limb. The Roux limb is created from a distal stump of the jejunum divided at about 30 to 50 cm distal to the ligament of Trietz [15]. The proximal stump then is anastomosed as entero-enterostomy to the Roux limb. The point of anastomosis dictates the length of the Roux limb. Even though RYGB is considered a gold-standard of gastric bypass procedure, this technique could be modified in numerous ways, such as variation in size of gastric pouch and gastrojejunostomy, length of the Roux limb, and method to create the gastric pouch [16]. RYGB has been shown to result in long-term and sustained weight loss in about 70% of patients [17]. Compared with pure restrictive procedures, RYGB has been shown to be more effective in terms of absolute amount and maintenance of weight loss [9,18–20].

Jejunoileal bypass merits mentioning even though the procedure no longer is performed because of the occurrence of fatal complications following the surgery. There were many patients, however, who had this operation and could remain subjected to its long-term complications. In this type of surgery, the jejunum was divided at 35 cm distal to the ligament of Treitz, and the proximal stump was anastomosed in an end-to-side manner to the terminal ileum, about 10 cm from the ileocecal valve [7]. About 300 to 500 cm of bowel was bypassed in this procedure. Jejunoileal bypass was popular and remained standard procedure for about 15 to 20 years but was found later to be associated with fatal hepatic failure and cirrhosis in most patients. Many patients also developed an autoimmune process causing fever, joint pain, and cutaneous eruption. Other complications included severe protein malnutrition, calcium oxalate nephropathy, electrolyte imbalance, severe vitamin and mineral deficiencies, diarrhea, bacterial overgrowth, and osteoporosis [21]. The procedure eventually was abandoned.

Complications after bariatric surgery could be perioperative, short-term (within the first year) or long-term [10]. The most common early perioperative complication is leakage of anastomosis [21], followed by obstruction and pulmonary embolism. Short-term complications include mainly issues related to weight loss and gall stone formation. Other commonly seen problems in this period include gastrointestinal (GI) symptoms such as nausea, vomiting, dumping syndrome, diarrhea, food intolerance, dehydration, and anastomotic ulcers [10,22].

Some GI symptoms will be focused on here, because they are related to the occurrence of neuromuscular complications after the surgery. Nausea and vomiting are the most common complaints after bariatric surgery [21]. These symptoms are seen more often in patients who have undergone restrictive procedures [10]. A very common cause is noncompliance to the recommended diet regimen after surgery [21]. This includes eating too fast, too much food volume in each meal, eating a big chunk of meat, especially red meat and poultry, and inadequate chewing. It is very important to rule out surgical complications such as stoma or outlet obstruction in patients who present with progressive vomiting or sudden intolerance to all types of food [22]. Dietary recommendations to prevent vomiting includes chewing thoroughly, eating meals slowly (longer than 20 minutes), small meal volume (less than 45 mL), and avoidance of meat in case of meat intolerance [21]. Dumping syndrome is seen more commonly after a combined procedure such as RYGB or in some patients who had malabsorptive procedures such as BPD [13,23]. The symptoms start in these patients soon after taking in a diet with high sugar content [21]. The symptoms of dumping syndrome can be divided into two phases, early and late, and have both GI and vasomotor, or autonomic, symptoms [10]. GI symptoms include nausea, abdominal cramps, and diarrhea. Vasomotor symptoms consist of tremulousness, profuse sweating, lightheadedness, flushing, and syncope [21,23]. The early phase of dumping syndrome is caused by rapid transit of hyperosmolar food content, especially food rich in carbohydrates, into the small intestine, causing fluid shift from the vascular space into the GI tract [24]. Another factor precipitating the early phase is increased surge of enteropeptides. The late phase of dumping syndrome occurs about 1 to 3 hours after eating and is caused by reactive hyperinsulinemic hypoglycemia [24]. Management includes avoiding food high in sugar or fat, small meals, and use of somatostatin or its analog [22,24]. Diarrhea is frequently seen after RYGB and BPD. After RYGB, diarrhea can be a presentation of dumping syndrome [16]. After BPD, diarrhea, malodorous stool, and gas occur mainly as a result of fat malabsorption and are seen less frequently when the common' limb is 100 cm [14]. The other causes of diarrhea include infection, bacterial overgrowth, and food or lactose intolerance [10].

Metabolic complications after bariatric surgery and its neurological disorders

Because the aim of bariatric surgery is to significantly reduce amount of food intake and alter the route of food absorption, metabolic complications, particularly from protein–calorie malnutrition and vitamin and mineral deficiencies tend to occur [25]. The type and severity of metabolic complications depend on the type of surgery. Of note is that about 20% to 30% of obese patients who underwent bariatric surgery were found to have micronutrient deficiency even before surgery [25]. This mandates a careful preoperative evaluation of the nutritional status [26]. The mechanisms by which neurologic injury occur after bariatric surgery are related mostly to metabolic or nutritional complications. Detailed general discussion about all nutritional deficiency is beyond the scope of this article. Only the nutrient deficiency that potentially causes neuromuscular complications after bariatric surgery will be focused on here. These are vitamin B12 (cobalamin), vitamin B1(thiamine), copper, calcium and vitamin D, folate, and vitamin B6 (pyridoxine).

Vitamin B12 is essential in DNA synthesis, being a cofactor for folate-dependent methionine synthase and mitochondrial–β-oxidation of fatty acids, being a cofactor for methylmalonyl coA mutase [27]. It is also probably essential for neurologic function, because the deficiency may cause both central and peripheral neurological disorders [28]. After bariatric surgery, vitamin B12 deficiency occurs commonly. The prevalence is from 12% [29] to 70% [30]. Mechanisms of deficiency include reduced acidity in the stomach pouch, meat intolerance, and reduced intrinsic factor secretion

after bariatric surgery [21]. Vitamin B12 deficiency is seen most frequently after RYGB and BPD [12]. It occurs more frequently in patients who develop meat intolerance and nonvitamin users after the surgery [31]. B12 deficiency causes hematological, GI, and neurological disorders. The most well-known neurological disorder arising from B12 deficiency is subacute combined degeneration of spinal cord. After bariatric surgery, parenteral (subcutaneous or intramuscular) administration of 1000 μg once a month is recommended for B12 supplementation [32], even though oral B12 supplementation at the dose of 350 μg daily has been reported to be effective [33]. Interestingly, even though low serum levels of vitamin B12 are common after bariatric surgery, most cases are asymptomatic [34,35]. Subacute combined degeneration from B12 deficiency has been reported after partial gastrectomy from the other indications [36] and has been reported after bariatric surgery only recently [37].

Vitamin B1 plays an important role in both metabolic and nerve functions, including acetylcholine receptor clustering [28] and acetylcholine biosynthesis [38]. Vitamin B1 is reabsorbed predominantly in duodenum and jejunum, through a carrier-mediated transport (at lower intakes) and passive diffusion (at higher intakes) [39]. Only a small amount is stored in the body, mainly in the muscles and the rest in heart, liver, kidneys, and the nervous tissue [38]. In bariatric surgery, reduced absorption of vitamin B1 occurs from reduced acid production from stomach and, most importantly, following prolonged and severe nausea and vomiting [40–42] The prevalence of thiamine deficiency after bariatric surgery is unknown but is associated mostly with VBG, where reduced food intake is the main cause [12]. Vitamin B1 deficiency causes peripheral (beriberi) and central (Wernicke's encephalopathy) neurological disorders [39]. In Western populations, B1 deficiency manifesting as Wernicke's encephalopathy and beriberi is very rare, seen mainly in alcoholics. On the other hand, beriberi is seen predominantly in Asian populations, especially in people who eat milled rice and have high carbohydrate intake but low meat intake. This difference in clinical predisposition is of unclear cause, but different genetic background may play a role [39]. Beriberi, however, has been reported in adolescents who underwent RYGB [43]. It is very important to recognize the syndrome, because prompt treatment results in dramatic improvement, and late treatment can result in permanent neurologic sequelae. The recommended treatment is immediate intravenous administration of thiamine 100 mg, followed by 100 mg intramuscularly daily for 5 days and oral maintenance permanently [28]. Intravenous glucose without thiamine can precipitate Wernicke's encephalopathy in a severely malnourished patient. To confirm the diagnosis of vitamin B1 deficiency, measurement of erythrocyte transketolase activity is the most reliable [39]. The prevalence of Wernicke's encephalopathy after bariatric surgery is unknown. Wernicke's encephalopathy after bariatric surgery has been reviewed recently [44]. The onset was mostly 4 to 12 weeks after surgery. The syndrome was seen after both restrictive and combined

procedures. Vomiting was the most common predisposing factor. Most patients had the clinical triad of the syndrome. Treatment with parenteral thiamine results in a complete recovery in most patients.

Copper deficiency recently has emerged as a cause of neurological disorders following gastric surgery [45]. Copper absorption into intestinal mucosa requires copper transporters (Ctr1 copper transporter and DCT-1) [46]. It then is transported to ATP7A to be exported from the intestinal cells into the circulation. Clinically, copper deficiency causes hematologic and neurologic manifestations [47]. Neurological symptoms start subacutely in the form of myeloneuropathy. The frequency of copper deficiency after bariatric surgery remains unknown. So far, there has been no general recommendation regarding copper supplement after bariatric surgery. The clinical syndrome, however, needs to be recognized and the deficiency corrected promptly if it happens.

Calcium and vitamin D have a major function in maintaining bone health in the human body [48,49]. Vitamin D works through its active form, 1, $25(OH)_2D$. The primary action of 1, 25 $(OH)_2$ D is to promote intestinal absorption of calcium and phosphorus through the small intestine. This reaction is regulated by parathyroid hormone. Moreover, calcium is also important in nerve and muscle functions [12]. Calcium is absorbed mainly in the duodenum and proximal jejunum, whereas vitamin D is absorbed mainly in the jejunum and ileum [29]. After RYGB and BPD, calcium and vitamin D deficiency predictably occurs. Possible causes include bypassing the duodenum and proximal jejunum, food intolerance, and fat malabsorption. The frequencies of calcium and vitamin D deficiencies were reportedly 10% and 50%, respectively, after RYGB [50]. The deficiency results in osteoporosis and osteomalacia. Neurologically, osteomalacia and vitamin D deficiency long have been known to be associated with proximal myopathy (osteomalacic myopathy) [51]. Measurement of serum vitamin D, urine calcium, serum bone alkaline phosphatase (BAP), and serum parathyroid hormone (PTH) levels would help establishing the diagnosis. In general, serum vitamin D and 24-hour urine calcium are decreased (total 25–OH D less than 15 ng/mL), and the levels of BAP and PTH are elevated [35]. Treatment with vitamin D supplement results in definite improvement in strength and pain. [51,52] The recommended vitamin D supplementation after bariatric surgery is to administer 50,000 IU of vitamin D3 (cholecalciferol) or vitamin D2 (ergocalciferol) once per week [35]. A case of osteomalacic myopathy after jejunoileal bypass has been reported [53].

Folate or folic acid consists of pterin linked to p-aminobezoic acid. The most common tissue form of folic acid is methyl-tetrahydrofolate (methyl-THF) [28]. Vitamin B12 acts as a coenzyme in the conversion of methyl-THF to THF, the biologically active form. B12 deficiency then can cause folate deficiency [21]. Folate is absorbed mainly at the proximal intestine, mediated by a saturable, specific carrier [27,28]. Absorption by diffusion, however, may also occur at high concentrations [27]. After bariatric surgery, folate deficiency occurs as a result of reduced food intake and reduced

gastric acid secretion that facilitates folate absorption [21]. The incidence could be as high as 35% [38]. Folate deficiency after bariatric surgery may present with megaloblastic anemia [54] or could be asymptomatic [38]. Neurologically, folate deficiency has been reported to be associated with peripheral neuropathy [55,56] or neuropsychiatric disorders [57]. In some cases, the clinical features of subacute combined degeneration have been observed [55]. The incidence of neurological complications is very low, however, and the association of these neurologic manifestations to folate deficiency has been debated [28,32]. The recommended dose of folate supplement after bariatric surgery is 1 mg/d [21,29].

Vitamin B6 consists of three main active derivatives: pyridoxal, pyridoxine, and pyridoxamine [27]. The incidence of B6 deficiency after bariatric surgery is about 17% [58] Neurological disorders resulting from B6 deficiency after bariatric surgery never have been reported, however.

Neuromuscular complications after bariatric surgery

Most neuromuscular complications after bariatric surgery were reported in case reports or case series. A recent review showed that the most commonly reported neurologic complications were peripheral neuropathy, followed by Wernicke's encephalopathy [59]. The most commonly reported muscle disorder after bariatric surgery is rhabdomyolysis.

There have been two large studies on the neurologic complications after bariatric surgery. The first one was by Abarbanel and colleagues [60], and the second one was by Thaisetthawatkul and colleagues [61]. In the first study, 500 patients who underwent bariatric surgery (457 RYGB and 43 gastroplasty) were studied from 1979 to 1984. Twenty three patients developed different neurologic syndromes at about 3 to 20 months (mean 8 months) postoperatively. The most common neurologic disorders were various forms of peripheral neuropathy (one acute polyneuropathy, two burning feet syndrome, 12 chronic polyneuropathy, and two meralgia paresthetica). The other neurologic complications included myotonic syndrome, posterolateral myelopathy, and Wernicke-Korsakoff encephalopathy. Most patients who developed neurologic complications had complaints of protracted nausea and vomiting after surgery. Of note is that in this study, burning foot syndrome responded well to thiamine administration. Subacute or chronic polyneuropathy cases did not respond dramatically to multivitamin supplement or increased calorie intake, and cases of posterolateral myelopathy had normal B12 studies. As expected, cases of Wernicke's encephalopathy responded well to thiamine administration [60]. The second study looked particularly at the association of peripheral neuropathy and bariatric surgery. The main questions are whether:

- peripheral neuropathy occurs more frequently after bariatric surgery than other abdominal surgery

- If so, what types of neuropathy there are
- What the risk factors are

The study consisted of 425 patients who had bariatric surgery. Of these, 71(16%) patients developed peripheral neuropathy. Three hundred age- and gender-matched obese patients who underwent open cholecystectomy were recruited as a control group, and in that group, only four (3%) patients developed peripheral neuropathy postoperatively, significantly less than the bariatric group. This suggested that the occurrence of peripheral neuropathy after bariatric surgery should not result from the fact that the patients had an open abdominal surgery. Three main clinical syndromes of postbariatric peripheral neuropathy were defined in the second study [61]. These were predominantly sensory neuropathy, mononeuropathy, and radiculoplexus neuropathy. The clinical features of predominantly sensory polyneuropathy group consisted of symmetrical sensory symptoms and signs of insidious onset and chronic progression. Both positive and negative sensory symptoms were present. Only a small number of patients developed distal weakness in the lower limbs. Autonomic symptoms such as constipation, lightheadedness, or syncope and impotence were observed. Electrophysiologic study in this group of patients showed features of axonal sensorimotor polyneuropathy. A small number of patients had electrodiagnostic features of a small fiber neuropathy. In the mononeuropathy group, the most common was median mononeuropathy across the wrist (carpal tunnel syndrome), followed by radial neuropathy, ulnar neuropathy, lateral femoral cutaneous neuropathy (meralgia paresthetica), peroneal neuropathy, sciatic neuropathy, and greater occipital neuropathy. In the radiculoplexus neuropathy group, both upper limb involvement and lower limb involvement were observed. The clinical features were in general similar to cases seen in nonsurgical setting. In that study, risk factors of developing neuropathy after bariatric surgery included:

Rapid weight loss

- Prolonged GI symptoms (nausea and vomiting, dumping syndrome, and diarrhea) after surgery
- Not attending the nutritional clinic after surgery
- Malnutrition state (reduced serum albumin and transferrin postoperatively)
- Having postoperative surgical complications requiring hospitalization
- Having jejunoileal bypass

Interestingly, in subgroup analysis, most of the risk factors identified were related to the polyneuropathy group, suggesting that the polyneuropathy group is more related to nutritional factors and status than mononeuropathy and radiculoplexus neuropathy groups. The study, however, also observed active axonal degeneration and significant inflammation in four sural nerve biopsies done in patients who had predominantly sensory polyneuropathy. Even though the polyneuropathy group had risk factors related to nutritional status, no specific nutritional deficiency was identified in that study [61]. Vitamin B12 and folate levels were not different between the group of patients who developed and who did not develop neuropathy after surgery. The study emphasized the importance of having adequate nutritional support after surgery.

Some important points are worth mentioning for peripheral neuropathy after bariatric surgery. Peripheral neuropathy is the most common neurologic complication reported after bariatric surgery. The etiology of most cases of polyneuropathy, however, was unclear, even though postoperative malnutrition status seems to play a role in pathogenesis [61]. Many case reports or series showed that nutritional and multivitamin supplements may help in improving symptoms of polyneuropathy in these patients [62–65]. Thiamine also has been shown to be an important cause of polyneuropathy in patients undergoing gastrectomy (for other indications than morbid obesity) [66]. in the previously mentioned large study of bariatric patients, however, nutritional and vitamin supplement seemed not to be helpful in cases of subacute or chronic polyneuropathy [60]. In many cases, specific nutritional deficiency was not found [61], and common nutritional deficiency, such as vitamin B12 and folate deficiency were not the causes of polyneuropathy. In some of these cases, a significant degree of inflammation was found in a sural nerve biopsy [61]. The cause of these inflammatory responses remains unclear. In patients who have diabetic or non diabetic radiculoplexus neuropathy, inflammatory microvasculitis has been shown to play an important role in pathogenesis [67,68]. These disorders often are associated with significant weight loss at the time of the onset. Because significant weight loss seems to be a common factor here, it raises the question whether rapid, significant weight loss and, in case of bariatric surgery, malnutrition, can induce abnormal immune response somehow, causing inflammatory neuropathy. This question remains unanswered. Moreover, it is also unclear if immune therapy alone will be adequate in treating postbariatric polyneuropathy patients who have inflammation in a nerve biopsy. Postoperative nutritional management and management of postoperative surgical complications remain very important [61]. Because most patients who developed peripheral neuropathy reported prolonged and severe nausea and vomiting and other GI symptoms [60,61], patients who have these symptoms should be the target for these measures to hopefully prevent the occurrence of peripheral neuropathy. The second important point to mention is the recognition of copper deficiency that recently has emerged as a cause of myeloneuropathy following gastric surgery [45]. Theis entity has been increasingly reported [69–71]. Because this condition is potentially manageable, it is very important to recognize it early to prevent further progression. The third important point to mention is about mononeuropathies following bariatric surgery. Many cases of mononeuropathies, especially peroneal neuropathy, have been reported after weight loss [72–74] and bariatric surgery [75]. The mechanism likely is related to loss of fat pad to protect the nerve from compression [75]. It is not, therefore, surprising that many cases of mononeuropathies were reported after bariatric surgery, most commonly lateral femoral cutaneous neuropathy or meralgia paresthetica [59]. The cause remains unclear but was thought to be from compression by Gomez retractor [76], even though it still happens when the questioned retractor is not used [77]. Meralgia paresthetica also has been reported after the other types of surgery such as coronary bypass surgery [78] or posterior spine surgery [79]. Because meralgia paresthetica occurs very soon after bariatric surgery before weight loss happens [77], it is seen more often in obese individuals [80], and it also is seen more in obese patients undergoing the other types of surgery [79]. It is likely that meralgia paresthetica after bariatric surgery results from the nerve compression from obesity itself. Most cases resolve spontaneously in a few months after surgery [78,79]. Of note is that in the study by Thaisetthawatkul colleagues, median mononeuropathy across the wrist or carpal tunnel syndrome was the most common mononeuropathy seen after bariatric surgery [61]. The reason remains unclear, because carpal tunnel syndrome is known to have positive correlation to increased BMI and obesity [81,82]. It is possible that rapid weight loss makes the nerve more susceptible to compression [61].

Postoperative rhabdomyolysis increasingly has been recognized as a myopathic complication after bariatric surgery, from both open [83] and laparoscopic [84] surgery. Rhabdomyolysis is a clinical and biochemical syndrome characterized by skeletal muscle necrosis and release of intracellular muscle content into the circulation [85]. It may result in asymptomatic elevation of muscle enzyme or life-threatening conditions such as renal failure, electrolyte imbalance, or compartmental syndrome. The incidences vary from 1.4% [86] to 26% [87]. Typically, serum creatine kinase (CPK) will peak and reach maximum level on the first day postoperatively [87,88]. Most authors used postoperative CPK greater than 1000 IU/L as a criteria to diagnose postbariatric rhabdomyolysis [87–89], and CPK level in rhabdomyolysis could be as high as 50,000 [89]. Risk factors include massive obesity and prolonged operative time [87,88]. Renal failure requiring hemodialysis develops in about 40% of patients who have rhabdomyolysis [89]. Preventive measures consisting of aggressive fluid replacement, forced diuresis, and urine alkalinization when the CPK rises above 5,000 IU/L have been shown to prevent renal failure [88]. Other preventive measures include attention to intraoperative padding to pressure points, frequent intraoperative and postoperative positioning of the patients, and limiting the duration of the operation [90,91].

Summary

Neuromuscular complications after bariatric surgery increasingly are recognized as the number of surgeries performed is increasing. Peripheral neuropathy is the most commonly reported neurologic disorders after bariatric surgery. Risk factors of polyneuropathy after bariatric surgery are related to postoperative nutritional status, rate of weight loss, and postoperative surgical complications, underscoring the importance of optimal surgical technique and adequate and efficient nutritional management after surgery. Common nutritional deficiency syndrome that involves neuromuscular system, such as thiamine, cobalamin, folate, pyridoxine and vitamin D deficiencies, needs to be recognized and treated promptly. Copper deficiency recently has emerged as cause of a neurologic disorder after GI surgery. Its clinical syndrome needs to be recognized so that treatment can be started earlier to prevent further progression. Rhabdomyolysis is another important postoperative complication that can be life-threatening. Early recognition and aggressive measures to help prevent renal failure are important.

References

[1] Latifi R, Sugarman H. Surgical treatment of obesity. In: Eckel R, editor. Obesity: mechanisms and clinical management. Philadelphia: Lippincott Williams & Wilkins; 2003. p. 503–22.

[2] Eckel R. Obesity: a disease or a physiologic adaptation for survival? In: Eckel R, editor. Obesity: mechanisms and clinical management. Philadelphia: Lippincott Williams & Wilkins; 2003. p. 3–30.

[3] Wing R, Phelan S. Behavioral treatment of obesity: strategies to improve outcome and predictors of success. In: Eckel R, editor. Obesity: mechanisms and clinical management. Philadelphia: Lippincott Williams & Wilkins; 2003. p. 415–35.

[4] Drewnowski A, Warren-Mears V. Nutrition and obesity. In: Eckel R, editor. Obesity: mechanisms and clinical management. Philadelphia: Lippincott Williams & Wilkins; 2003. p. 4436–48.

[5] Bray G. Treatment of obesity with drugs in the new millennium. In: Eckel R, editor. Obesity: mechanisms and clinical management. Philadelphia: Lippincott Williams & Wilkins; 2003. p. 449–75.

[6] National Institute of Health Consensus Development Conference Panel. Gastrointestinal surgery for severe obesity. Ann Intern Med 1991;115(12):956–61.

[7] Martin L. The evolution of surgery for morbid obesity. In: Martin L, editor. Obesity surgery. New York: McGraw-Hill; 2004. p. 15–48.

[8] Salem L, Jensen C, Flum D. Are bariatric surgical outcomes worth their cost?: a systematic review. J Am Coll Surg 2005;200(2):270–8.

[9] Sjostrom L, Lindroos A, Peltonen M, et al. Lifestyle, diabetes, and cardiovascular risk factors 10 years after bariatric surgery. N Engl J Med 2004;351:2683–93.

[10] Abell T, Minocha A. Gastrointestinal complications of bariatric surgery: diagnosis and therapy. Am J Med Sci 2006;331(4):214–8.

[11] Martin L. Gastric restrictive procedures: gastroplasties and bands. In: Martin L, editor. Obesity surgery. New York: McGraw-Hill; 2004. p. 193–211.

[12] Malinowski S. Nutritional and metabolic complications of bariatric surgery. Am J Med Sci 2006;331(4):219–25.

[13] Monteforte M, Turkelson C. Bariatric surgery for morbid obesity. Obes Surg 2000;10: 391–401.

[14] Marceau P, Biron S, Hould F, et al. Current malabsorptive procedures: biliopancreatic diversion. In: Martin L, editor. Obesity surgery. New York: McGraw-Hill; 2004. p. 227–42.

[15] Kendrick M, Dakin G. Surgical approach to obesity. Mayo Clin Proc 2006;81(Suppl 10): S18–24.

[16] Pories W, Roth J. Gastric bypass. In: Martin L, editor. Obesity surgery. New York: McGraw-Hill; 2004. p. 213–25.

[17] Balsinger B, Kennedy F, Abu-Lebdeh H, et al. Prospective evaluation of Roux-en-Y gastric bypass as primary operation for medically complicated obesity. Mayo Clin Proc 2000;75: 673–80.

[18] Linner J. Comparative effectiveness of gastric bypass and gastroplasty: a clinical study. Arch Surg 1982;117:695–700.

[19] Maggard M, Shugarman L, Suttorp M, et al. Meta-analysis: surgical treatment of obesity. Ann Intern Med 2005;142:547–59.

[20] Buchwald H, Avidor Y, Braunwald E, et al. Bariatric surgery: a systematic review and meta-analysis. JAMA 2004;292:1724–37.

[21] Ukleja A, Stone R. Medical and gastroenterologic management of the postbariatric surgery patient. J Clin Gastroenterol 2004;38:312–21.

[22] Parkes E. Nutritional management of patients after bariatric surgery. Am J Med Sci 2006; 331(4):207–13.

[23] Martin L. Managing postoperative complications after bariatric surgery. In: Martin L, editor. Obesity surgery. New York: McGraw-Hill; 2004. p. 259–74.

[24] Vecht J, Masclee A, Lamers C. The dumping syndrome. Current insights into pathophysiology, diagnosis, and treatment. Scand J Gastroenterol 1997;32(Suppl 223):21–7.

[25] Mason M, Jalagani H, Vinik A. Metabolic complications of bariatric surgery: diagnosis and management issues. Gastroenterol Clin North Am 2005;34:25–33.

[26] Collazo-Clavell M, Clark M, McAlpine D, et al. Assessment and preparation of patients for bariatric surgery. Mayo Clin Proc 2006;81(Suppl 10):S11–17.

[27] Shane B. Folic acid, vitamin B12, and vitamin B6. In: Stipanuk M, editor. Biochemical, physiological, molecular aspects of human nutrition. St. Louis (MO): Saunders Elsevier; 2006. p. 693–732.

[28] Kumar N. Nutritional neuropathies. Neurol Clin 2007;(25):209–55.

[29] Alvarez-Leite J. Nutritional deficiency secondary to bariatric surgery. Curr Opin Clin Nutr Metab Care 2004;7:569–75.

[30] Fujioka K. Follow-up of nutritional and metabolic problems after bariatric surgery. Diabetes Care 2005;28:481–4.

[31] Avinoah E, Ovnat A, Charuzi I. Nutritional status seven years after Roux-en-Y gastric bypass surgery. Surgery 1992;111:137–42.

[32] McMahon M, Sarr M, Clark M, et al. Clinical management after bariatric surgery: value of a multidisciplinary approach. Mayo Clin Proc 2006;81(Suppl 10):S34–45.

[33] Rhode B, Tamin H, Gilfix B, et al. Treatment of vitamin B12 deficiency after gastric surgery for severe obesity. Obes Surg 1995;5:154–8.

[34] Schilling R, Gohdes P, Hardie G. Vitamin B12 deficiency after gastric bypass surgery for obesity. Ann Intern Med 1984;101:501–2.

[35] Brolm R, Gorman J, Gorman R, et al. Are vitamin B12 and folate deficiency clinically important after Roux-en-Y gastric bypass? J Gastrointest Surg 1998;2:436–42.

[36] Roos D. Neurological complications in patients with impaired vitamin B12 absorption following partial gastrectomy. Acta Neurol Scand 1978;(Suppl 69):1–77.

[37] Juhasz-Pocsine K, Rudnicki S, Archer R, et al. Neurologic complications of gastric bypass surgery for morbid obesity. Neurology 2007;68:1843–50.

[38] McCormick D. Niacin, riboflavin and thiamin. In: Stipanuk M, editor. Biochemical, physiological, molecular aspects of human nutrition. St. Louis (MO): Saunders Elsevier; 2006. p. 665–92.

[39] Phuapradit P. Vitamin deficiencies, intoxications and gastrointestinal disorders. In: Swash M, Oxbury J, editors. Clinical neurology. New York: Churchill Livingstone; 1991. p. 1695–710.

[40] Foster D, Falah M, Kadom N, et al. Wernicke's encephalopathy after bariatric surgery: losing more than just weight. Neurology 2005;65:1987.

[41] Nautiyal A, Singh S, Alaimo D, et al. Wernicke's encephalopathy—an emerging trend after bariatric surgery. Am J Med 2004;117:804–5.

[42] Seehra H, MacDermott N, Lascelles R, et al. Wernicke's encephalopathy after vertical banded gastroplasty for morbid obesity. BMJ 1996;312:434.

[43] Towbin A, Inge T, Garcia V, et al. Beriberi after gastric bypass surgery in adolescence. J Pediatr 2004;145:263–7.

[44] Singh S, Kumar A. Wernicke's encephalopathy after obesity surgery. Neurology 2007;68: 1–5.

[45] Kumar N, McEvoy K, Ahlskog E. Myelopathy due to copper deficiency following gastrointestinal surgery. Arch Neurol 2003;60:1782–5.

[46] Grider A. Zinc, copper and manganese. In: Stipanuk M, editor. Biochemical, physiological, molecular aspects of human nutrition. St. Louis (MO): Saunders Elsevier; 2006. p. 1043–67.

[47] Kumar N, Crum B, Petersen R, et al. Copper deficiency myelopathy. Arch Neurol 2004;61: 762–6.

[48] Holick. Vitamin D. In: Stipanuk M, editor. Biochemical, physiological, molecular aspects of human nutrition. St. Louis (MO): Saunders Elsevier; 2006. p. 863–83.

[49] Wood R. Calcium and phosphorus. In: Stipanuk M, editor. Biochemical, physiological, molecular aspects of human nutrition. St. Louis (MO): Saunders Elsevier; 2006. p. 863–83.

[50] Shah M, Simha V, Garg A. Review: long-term impact of bariatric surgery on body weight, comorbidities, and nutritional status. J Clin Endocrinol Metab 2006;91:4223–31.

[51] Smith R, Stern G. Myopathy, osteomalacia, and hyperparathryroidism. Brain 1967;90(3): 593–602.

[52] Russell J. Osteomalacic myopathy. Muscle Nerve 1994;17:578–80.

[53] Franck W, Hoffman G, Davis J, et al. Osteomalacia and weakness complicating jejunoileal bypass. J Rheumatol 1979;6(1):51–6.

[54] Amaral J, Thompson W, Caldwell M, et al. Prospective hematologic evaluation of gastric exclusion surgery for morbid obesity. Ann Surg 1985;201(2):186–93.

[55] Botez M, Peyronnard JM, Bachevalier J, et al. Polyneuropathy and folate deficiency. Arch Neurol 1978;35:581–4.

[56] Manzoor M, Runce J. Folate-responsive neuropathy: report of 10 cases. BMJ 1976;1: 1176–8.

[57] Shorvon S, Carney M, Chanarin I, et al. The neuropsychiatry of megaloblastic anemia. BMJ 1980;281:1036–8.

[58] Clements R, Katasani V, Palepu R, et al. Incidence of vitamin deficiency after laparoscopic Roux-en-Y gastric bypass in a university hospital setting. Am Surg 2006;72(12):1196–202.

[59] Koffman B, Greenfield J, Ali I, et al. Neurologic complications after surgery for obesity. Muscle Nerve 2006;33:166–76.

[60] Abarbanel J, Berginer V, Osimani A, et al. Neurologic complications after gastric restriction surgery for morbid obesity. Neurology 1987;37:196–200.

[61] Thaisetthawatkul P, Collazo-Clavell M, Sarr G, et al. A controlled study of peripheral neuropathy after bariatric surgery. Neurology 2004;63:1462–70.

[62] Feit H, Glasberg M, Ireton C, et al. Peripheral neuropathy and starvation after gastric partitioning for morbid obesity. Ann Intern Med 1982;96:453–5.

[63] Maryniak O. Severe peripheral neuropathy following gastric bypass surgery for morbid obesity. Can Med Assoc J 1984;131:119–20.

[64] Nakamura K, Reilly L. Polyneuropathy following gastric bypass surgery. Am J Med 2003; 115:679–80.

[65] Chaves L, Faintuch J, Kahwage S, et al. A cluster of polyneuropathy and Wernicke-Korsakoff syndrome in a bariatric unit. Obes Surg 2002;12:328–34.

[66] Koike H, Misu K, Hattori N, et al. Postgastrectomy polyneuropathy with thiamine deficiency. J Neurol Neurosurg Psychiatry 2001;71:357–62.

[67] Dyck P, Windebank A. Diabetic and nondiabetic lumbosacral radiculoplexus neuropathies: new insights into pathophysiology and treatment. Muscle Nerve 2002;25:477–91.

[68] Dyck P, Norell J, Dyck P. Microvasculitis and ischemia in diabetic lumbosacral radiculo-plexus neuropathy. Neurology 1999;53:2113–21.

[69] Allred J, Aulino J. Hypocupremia-associated myelopathy. J Comput Assist Tomogr 2007; 31:157–9.

[70] Goodman B, Chong B, Patel A, et al. Copper deficiency myeloneuropathy resembling B12 deficiency: partial resolution of MR imaging findings with copper supplementation. AJNR Am J Neuroradiol 2006;27(10):2112–4.

[71] Tan J, Burns D, Jones H. Severe ataxia, myelopathy, and peripheral neuropathy due to acquired copper deficiency in a patient with history of gastrectomy. JPEN J Parenter Enteral Nutr 2006;30(5):446–50.

[72] Cruz-Martinez A, Arpa J, Palau F. Peroneal neuropathy after weight loss. J Peripher Nerv Syst 2000;5:101–5.

[73] Rubin D, Kimmel D, Cascino T. Outcome of peroneal neuropathies in patients with systemic malignant disease. Cancer 1998;83:1602–6.

[74] Ishii K, Tamaoka S, Matsuno S, et al. isolated peroneal nerve palsy complicating weight loss due to anterior pituitary hypofunction. Eur J Neurol 2003;10:187–8.

[75] Elias W, Pouratian N, Oskouian R, et al. Peroneal neuropathy following successful bariatric surgery. J Neurosurg 2006;105:631–5.

[76] Grace D. Meralgia paresthetica after gastroplasty for morbid obesity. Can J Surg 1987;30(1): 64–5.

[77] Macgregor A, Thoburn E. Maralgia paresthetica following bariatric surgery. Obes Surg 1999;9(4):364–8.

[78] Parsonnet V, Karasakalides A, Gielchinsky I, et al. Meralgia paresthetica after coronary bypass surgery. J Thorac Cardiovasc Surg 1991;101(2):219–21.

[79] Yang S, Wu C, Chen P. Postoperative meralgia paresthetica after posterior spine surgery: incidence, risk factors, and clinical outcomes. Spine 2005;30(18):E547–50.

[80] Seror P, Seror R. Meralgia paresthetica: clinical and electrophysiological diagnosis in 120 cases. Muscle Nerve 2006;33:650–4.

[81] Werner R, Albers J, Franzblau A, et al. The relationship between body mass index and the diagnosis of carpal tunnel syndrome. Muscle Nerve 1994;17:632–6.

[82] Stallings S, Kasdan M, Soergel T, et al. A case–control study of obesity as a risk factor for carpal tunnel syndrome in a population of 600 patients presenting for independent medical examination. J Hand Surg 1997;22:211–5.

[83] Collier B, Goreja M, Duke B. Postoperative rhabdomyolysis with bariatric surgery. Obes Surg 2003;13(6):941–3.

[84] Gorecki P, Cottam D, Ger R, et al. Lower extremity compartment syndrome following a laparoscopic Roux-en-Y gastric bypass. Obes Surg 2002;12(2):289–91.

[85] Gabow P, Kaehny W, Kelleher S. The spectrum of rhabdomyolysis. Medicine (Baltimore) 1982;61:141–52.

[86] Khurana R, Baudendistel T, Morgan E, et al. Postoperative rhabdomyolysis following laparoscopic gastric bypass in the morbidly obese. Arch Surg 2004;138:73–6.

[87] Langandre S, Arnalsteen L, Vallet B, et al. Predictive factors for rhabdomyolysis after bari-atric surgery. Obes Surg 2006;16:1365–70.

[88] Mognol P, Vignes S, Chosidow D, et al. Rhabdomyolysis after laparoscopic bariatric surgery. Obes Surg 2004;14:91–4.

[89] Faintuch J, de Clava R, Pajecki D, et al. Rhabdomyolysis after gastric bypass: severity and outcome patterns. Obes Surg 2006;16:1209–13.

[90] Bostanjian D, Anthone G, Hamoui N, et al. Rhabdomyolysis of gluteal muscles leading to renal failure: a potentially fatal complication of surgery in the morbidly obese. Obes Surg 2003;13(2):302–5.

[91] De Menezes Ettinger J, dos Santos Filho P, Azaro E, et al. Prevention of rhabdomyolysis in bariatric surgery. Obes Surg 2005;15(6):874–9.

ELSEVIER
SAUNDERS

Phys Med Rehabil Clin N Am
19 (2008) 125–148

PHYSICAL MEDICINE
AND REHABILITATION
CLINICS OF
NORTH AMERICA

Neuromuscular Complications
of Nutritional Deficiencies

Faren H. Williams, MD, MS, RD

*Department of Orthopedics and Physical Rehabilitation, University of Massachusetts
Memorial, 119 Belmont Street, Worcester, MA 01605-2982, USA*

Much is known about the effects of malnutrition on health in general. The British navy discovered that carrying limes on board would prevent the ravages of scurvy, a dreaded disease later found to be the result of vitamin C deficiency. For many nutrition deficiencies, a direct cause and effect of different symptoms and diseases has been established. These are known as primary nutritional deficiencies. Secondary deficiencies occur when the vitamin or nutrient requirement may be increased, such as in patients who have pernicious anemia who lack the intrinsic factor needed to absorb vitamin B12. Less well recognized are the effects of nutritional deficiencies on chronic disease, especially acute and chronic neuromuscular diseases. This article identifies some of the causative factors and provides the reader with a guideline for what to consider in the evaluation of individuals who have neuromuscular problems. The context of these disorders is best understood on a foundation of basic nutrition information.

Nutrition management principles

Food contains nutrients to support health and life. Good nutrition management ensures that individuals obtain all the substances in their diet to optimize health and provide a degree of satisfaction, because eating is one of the more powerful social activities. Almost every special occasion and most shared meals involve interaction with others. The subject of nutrition thus is intimately linked to one's psychologic sense of well being [1].

Individuals are well nourished, malnourished, or have overt nutritional deficiencies. Malnutrition has been defined as the lack of one or more nutrients in the diet. An abundance of food, increased longevity, and financial

E-mail addresses: williamf@ummhc.org; fhwmd@earthlink.net

resources to purchase different foods, however, has resulted in excessive and unbalanced nutrient intake.

Three conditions can result in suboptimal function secondary to malnutrition: (1) nutrition deficiency (undernutrition)—the result of insufficient intake of one or more nutrients to meet one's nutritional requirements for cellular health and optimal metabolism; (2) nutrient excess (overnutrition)—the result of excessive intake of one or more nutrients; and (3) nutrient imbalance—the result of consuming inadequate amounts of some nutrients and excessive amounts of others.

Malnutrition is a continuum in which body stores of nutrients are altered such that there is an imbalance, with some nutrients being depleted and others being excessive. If the imbalance persists, alterations of metabolism at the biochemical level and overt disease may result [1].

Nutrients

These are chemical substances that must be consumed to sustain life. They must also be consumed in the right proportions and in combination with other nutrients that enhance their absorption. The six general categories of these nutrients are water, proteins, carbohydrates, fats, vitamins, and minerals.

Water is the most basic compound essential for life, comprising more than 50% of the body mass. It is an integral part of cell structures and the basic medium for all body fluids. Proteins, carbohydrates, and fats all supply energy and have different functions in body composition, cell structure, and metabolic activity. The basic components of protein, amino acids, and of fats, essential fatty acids, cannot be synthesized in the body and need to be ingested from foods containing them. Optimal ratios of these three nutrients are essential for health and can be obtained from a balanced diet. Excessive consumption of one, such as protein, in the absence of adequate caloric intake from the other three nutrients can be harmful, because the liver needs to chemically remove the nitrogen to use it for energy. If the body's ability to excrete the nitrogen is exceeded, then ammonia may build up in the body. Excessive protein, fat, or carbohydrate is also converted to fat, leading to obesity, and skeletal muscle may be broken down to meet energy requirements if the caloric intake is inadequate [1].

Much is known about the deleterious effects of a diet inadequate in protein. Many individuals in the United States eat more than the recommended daily allowance for protein, yet certain population groups, such as those who have alcoholism, anorexia, illness of chronic disease, and the frail elderly who may already be malnourished, are at risk for developing protein calorie malnutrition. Epidemiologic studies have found a direct relationship between the risk for developing multiple sclerosis (MS) and dietary fat intake, especially animal fat [2]. One study found a correlation between a high intake of complex carbohydrates and MS [3].

Vitamins are either water- or fat-soluble, and many are cofactors for enzymatic reactions in metabolism. Fat-soluble and some water-soluble vitamins are stored in the body to varying extents, so they may not need to be ingested daily, but become depleted over time if the intake is less than adequate. Minerals are inorganic elements and include trace elements that are essential for health (Table 1).

Assessing nutritional status

Nutritional assessment means the gathering and interpretation of data from which the effect of disease, injury, other stressors, and nutritional intervention can be monitored over time. Nutritional screening identifies those patients who require more comprehensive nutritional assessment to determine the risk for malnutrition. The latter requires direct measurement of food intake for nutrients and calories, along with measures of clinical anthropometric, biochemical, and physiologic status. The extent of the assessment may vary depending on the person's problems and the nutritional goals. Known physical examination findings may alert the health care provider to the presence of specific nutritional deficiencies (Table 2).

Identifying nutritional risk

Nutritional risk that leads to malnutrition and hence neuromuscular complications involves many factors (Fig. 1). Certain population groups have higher risk. Young children have special nutrient requirements for growth, whereas the elderly have slower metabolism and decreased activity that lead them to require fewer calories but that doesn't decrease their need for specific nutrients. Those who are chronically ill have specific nutrition needs, and they may be on prolonged inadequate parenteral nutrition. Individuals who have eating disorders, anorexia and obesity, alcoholic patients who consume primarily alcohol, poor and homeless individuals who lack resources to purchase food, and those who have dysphagia, prolonged depression, or cognitive impairments may be at risk for inadequate intake of key nutrients. The elderly may have a unique combination of risk factors, including financial, social, multiple organ failure, decreased muscle mass, swallowing problems, and dementia, all of which may affect their ability to take in adequate nutrients and calories. As caloric intake decreases, it may be difficult to obtain essential nutrients. Still others who have malabsorption caused by diseases such as celiac sprue, Crohn disease, inflammatory bowel disease, or pernicious anemia are at risk. It is essential to consider multiple factors, including social, environmental, medical, and economic, which put the individual host at risk. When seeing an individual at follow-up, key questions include whether there has been any change in medical condition, cognition, mental health, physical activity, and ability to

Table 1
Vitamins and minerals

Nutrient	Major functions
Water-soluble vitamins	
Thiamin (vitamin B1)	Coenzyme in carbohydrate metabolism; nerve function
Riboflavin (vitamin B2)	Coenzyme in citric acid cycle, fat metabolism, and electron transport chain
Niacin (vitamin B3)	Coenzyme in citric acid cycle, fat metabolism, and electron transport chain
Biotin	Coenzyme in glucose production and fat synthesis
Pyridoxine	Coenzyme in protein metabolism, neurotransmitter, and hemoglobin synthesis
Pantothenic acid	Coenzyme in citric acid cycle and fat metabolism (synthesis and beta-oxidation)
Folate	Coenzyme in RNA and DNA synthesis
Vitamin B12	Coenzyme in folate metabolism, nerve function
Vitamin C	Collagen synthesis; hormone and neurotransmitter synthesis; antioxidant
Fat-soluble vitamins	
Vitamin A (retinoids and provitamin A carotenoids)	Vision; growth; cell differentiation; immunity; antioxidant
Vitamin D	Absorption of calcium and phosphorous; bone maintenance
Vitamin E	Antioxidant
Vitamin K	Blood clotting
Major minerals (<100 mg/day)	
Calcium	Bone and tooth structure; blood clotting; muscle contractions; nerve transmission
Phosphorous	Bone and tooth structure; intermediary metabolism; membrane structure; ATP
Sodium	Major extracellular cation; nerve transmission; regulates fluid balance
Potassium	Major intercellular cation; nerve–nerve transmission
Magnesium	Bone structure; enzyme function; nerve and muscle function; ATP
Chloride	Major extracellular anion; nerve transmission
Sulfur	Part of vitamins and amino acids; acid–base balance
Minor minerals (<20 mg/day)	
Iron	Part of hemoglobin and myoglobin; immunity
Cobalt	Part of vitamin B12
Manganese	Functions in carbohydrate and fat metabolism; superoxide dismutase
Molybdenum	Cofactor for several enzymes
Fluoride	Strengthens tooth enamel
Copper	Iron metabolism; superoxide dismutase; nerve and immune function; lipid metabolism; collagen
Zinc	Cofactor in hundreds of enzyme systems; protein synthesis; growth; immunity; superoxide dismutase; alcohol metabolism
Iodine	Synthesis of thyroid hormone
Selenium	Antioxidant function as component of glutathione peroxidase
Chromium	Glucose tolerance

Abbreviations: ATP, adenosine triphosphate; DNA, deoxyribonucleic acid; RNA, ribonucleic acid.

(*Adapted from* Williams FH, Hopkins B. Nutrition in physical medicine and rehabilitation. In: DeLisa J, Gans BM, Walsh NE, editors. Physical medicine and rehabilitation: principles and practices. Philadelphia: Lippincott-Raven; 2004. p. 1267–87; with permission.)

Table 2
Nutritional assessment: physical findings

Clinical findings	Possible nutritional causes
Hair	
Dyspigmentation (flat sign)	Protein deficiency
Easily plucked	Protein deficiency
Sparse	Protein, biotin, zinc deficiency
Corkscrew hairs	Vitamin C deficiency
Nails	
Spoon nails (koilonychia)	Iron deficiency
Brittle nails	Iron deficiency, excess vitamin A
Transverse ridging	Protein deficiency
Skin	
Scaling	Vitamin A, essential fatty acid, zinc deficiency
Follicular hyperkeratosis	Vitamin A deficiency
Purpura	Vitamin C, K deficiency
Yellow coloration	Excess carotene
Pellagrous dermatitis	Niacin deficiency
Cellophane appearance	Protein deficiency
Eyes	
Night blindness	Vitamin A deficiency
Bitot spots	Vitamin A deficiency
Papilledema	Vitamin A excess
Pale conjunctivae	Iron deficiency
Mouth	
Angular stomatitis	Riboflavin, niacin, pyridoxine deficiency
Cheilosis	Riboflavin, niacin, pyridoxine deficiency
Tongue	
Pale, atrophic	Iron deficiency
Atrophic lingual papillae	Riboflavin, niacin, folate, vitamin B12, protein, iron deficiency
Glossitis (scarlet)	Riboflavin, niacin, folate, vitamin B12, pyridoxine deficiency
Hypogeusia	Zinc deficiency
Gums	
Spongy, bleeding	Vitamin C deficiency
Musculoskeletal	
Beading of ribs	Vitamin D deficiency
Muscle wasting	Protein-calorie malnutrition
Tenderness	Vitamin C deficiency
Neurologic	
Confusion	Thiamin, niacin, vitamin B12 deficiency
Ophthalmoplegia	Thiamin, phosphorous deficiency
Peripheral neuropathy	Thiamin, pyridoxine, vitamin B12 deficiency
Tetany	Calcium deficiency
Other	
Cardiomegaly	Thiamine deficiency
Cardiomyopathy	Selenium deficiency
Hepatomegaly	Protein malnutrition
Edema	Protein, thiamin deficiency
Thyroid enlargement	Iodide deficiency

(*Adapted from* Williams FH, Hopkins B. Nutrition in physical medicine and rehabilitation. In: DeLisa J, Gans BM, Walsh NE, editors. Physical medicine and rehabilitation: principles and practices. Philadelphia: Lippincott-Raven; 2004. p. 1267–87; with permission.)

Has there been a change in any of the following?

1. Income   _____

2. Living Situation   _____

3. Source of Food   _____

4. Medical Condition   _____

5. Physical Activity   _____

6. Transportation   _____

7. Employment Status   _____

8. Eating Habits   _____

Fig. 1. Identifying nutritional risk. (*Adapted from* Williams FH, Hopkins B. Nutrition in physical medicine and rehabilitation. In: DeLisa J, Gans BM, Walsh NE, editors. Physical medicine and rehabilitation: principles and practices. Philadelphia: Lippincott-Raven; 2004. p. 1267–87; with permission.)

obtain or prepare food because of changes in income, employment status, transportation, or living situation. All of these factors determine one's overall eating habits and nutritional status (Fig. 2).

Neuromuscular disorders

For optimal functioning of the nervous system, one needs to have adequate intake of the water-soluble B-group vitamins—in particular, thiamine, niacin, pyridoxine, and vitamin B12, fat-soluble vitamins D and E, folic acid, copper, and zinc. Peripheral nerve problems and less frequently myopathy can occur because of deficiencies of one or more of these essential nutrients [1].

Thiamine deficiency

Thiamine deficiency is named "beriberi," the first identified human nutritional deficiency. Thiamine serves as a coenzyme in the metabolism of carbohydrates and branch chain amino acids. When there is inadequate thiamine, there is a decreased synthesis of high-energy phosphates, and lactate accumulates. There is a decreased level of alpha KGDH, a rate-limiting enzyme in the tricarboxylic acid cycle, that results in the decreased synthesis of amino acid neurotransmitters [4]. Vitamin B1 might have a role in nerve function involving acetylcholine receptor clustering [5] and acetylcholine biosynthesis [6].

Main food sources for vitamin B1 include meat (pork), cereals and grain products, legumes, and fruits [6]. Vitamin B1 is reabsorbed predominantly

Check if answer to question is yes. Nutrition risk increases as the number of checks increases.

1. Are you on a special diet? _____

2. Have you had a change in your eating habits? _____

3. Has your weight changed? _____

4. Do you have any cravings or desires for specific foods, liquids,or other substances to eat or drink? _____

5. Has your appetite changed? _____

6. Do you eat most of your food away from home? _____

7. Are you experiencing any of the following?

   a. Difficulty seeing at night? _____
   b. Dry skin or rashes? _____
   c. Nausea or vomiting? _____
   d. Constipation or diarrhea? _____
   e. Swelling of legs? _____
   f. Change if hair color, texture, or thickness (other than chemically or mechanically in duced by hair care? _____

   g. Yellow skin or eyes? _____
   h. Easy bruising? _____
   i. Swollen, tender joints? _____
   j. Poor healing of minor cuts or scratches? _____

8. Have you been ill or had surgery? _____

9. Are you taking any medicines or supplements?

10. Do you avoid any foods, liquids, or additives because of allergies or bad reactions? _____

Fig. 2. Determining overall eating habits and nutritional status. (*Adapted from* Williams FH, Hopkins B. Nutrition in physical medicine and rehabilitation. In: DeLisa J, Gans BM, Walsh NE, editors. Physical medicine and rehabilitation: principles and practices. Philadelphia: Lippincott-Raven; 2004. p. 1267–87; with permission.)

in the duodenum and jejunum through a carrier-mediated transport (at lower intakes) and passive diffusion (at higher intakes) [7]. This vitamin cannot be synthesized [8]; the half-life is 10 to 14 days, and the body stores are 30 to 100 mg. A deficiency thus could occur in as little as 6 to 8 weeks. One needs a continuous dietary supply, 1 to 1.5 mg per day. Alcoholic individuals who consume primarily hard liquor (beer has B vitamins) are prone to thiamine deficiency. Because of inadequate intake, liver stores are rapidly deleted and gastrointestinal absorption is impaired, because alcohol inhibits the transport of thiamine in the gastrointestinal tract and blocks the phosphorylation of thiamine to thiamine pyrophosphate (TPP). Individuals who have higher metabolic rates and those who are malnourished or who are on high-carbohydrate, low-protein diets with the main staple being milled rice have higher requirements. This includes high-risk patients participating in vigorous exercise with high-carbohydrate intake or those who are receiving IV glucose. Administration of IV glucose to a vitamin-depleted alcoholic patient or one at risk may precipitate a florid syndrome if supplementary vitamins are not provided [5].

The most vulnerable to a deficiency are the tissues with the highest turnover, caudal brain and cerebellum. Different types of deficiency are dry, wet, and infantile beriberi, with the dry form causing sensorimotor distal, axonal, peripheral neuropathy as noted by electrodiagnosis and sural nerve biopsy, leg cramps, muscle tenderness, and burning feet [9,10]. On clinical examination, one may find ankle and toe weakness with foot drop, decreased ankle jerks, and decreased fine motor and vibratory sense, with more generalized stocking/glove hypoesthesia, hypalgesia, and severe weakness later. Severe cases may also affect the phrenic and vagal nerves, and there may be associated autonomic neuropathy and tongue and facial weakness [11,12]. The neurologic changes often do not resolve completely with treatment.

Wet beriberi may cause pedal edema, high-output congestive heart failure, cardiac failure with lactic acidosis, and sensorimotor peripheral neuropathy, and it can become dry after diuresis. These symptoms respond dramatically to parenteral administration of thiamine. The infantile form, or Shoshin beriberi, bears little resemblance to the adult type and involves cardiac problems, aphonia, and a pseudomeningismus [13].

The most common central nervous system (CNS)-related neurologic problem in the alcoholic individual is Wernicke-Korsakoff syndrome. Wernicke encephalopathy (WE) is characterized by gait ataxia secondary to cerebellar dysfunction or polyneuropathy, confusion, and ocular palsies (with nystagmus lateral and conjugate gaze) [14,15]. There may be hypothermia, orthostatic hypotension, skin changes, truncal ataxia, features of liver disease, tongue redness, and an associated peripheral neuropathy in 80% of individuals. MRI reveals T2 enhancement around the third or fourth ventricle, periaqueductal midbrain, dorsal medial, thalami, and mammillary bodies [16] and hemorrhagic brainstem lesions that can cause sudden death [17]. Pathologic studies of the brains in fatal cases demonstrate necrotic or hemorrhagic lesions in many areas of the brainstem and brainstem nuclei. Wernicke encephalopathy may occur within 4 to 12 weeks after bariatric surgery as mentioned elsewhere in this issue, with most patients having the clinical triad mentioned [18]. Treatment with parenteral thiamine results in significant recovery, with the abnormal findings on MRI disappearing.

Korsakoff psychosis occurs after the ocular manifestations and encephalopathy subside and involves similar areas of the brain as Wernicke. The psychosis is characterized by anterograde amnesia, retrograde amnesia to a lesser extent, a disordered time sense, and confabulation in the later stages [5,19].

The erythrocyte transketolase activation is the preferred laboratory study to confirm a deficiency, because urine and serum do not reflect tissue stores well [20,21]. Treatment of thiamine deficiency is possible but may be precarious in at-risk patients.

They should receive parenteral thiamine before IV glucose or parenteral nutrition, because the IV glucose may consume what is there and may precipitate Wernicke encephalopathy.

To treat beriberi the patient needs 100 mg IV thiamine, then 100 mg intramuscular thiamine daily for 5 days, with a permanent oral maintenance dose of 50 to 100 mg [22]. The wet type improves rapidly, with clearing of symptoms within 24 hours to 1 week and improvement in sensory or motor symptoms within weeks to months [9].

With alcoholism-related neuropathy, the lipophilic form of thiamine should be used, 320 mg daily for 4 weeks, then 120 mg daily for another 3 weeks [23].

Response to WE treatment is variable for improvement in gait ataxia/memory, but the apathy and lethargy may improve over months [24].

Even with thiamine treatment, there may be 10% to 20% mortality. Some patients who have Korsakoff syndrome have impaired memory and learning long term.

A proximal myopathy with muscle weakness and myalgias may also be associated with a thiamine deficiency [25], because it decreases the production of ATP needed for muscle contraction. With less ATP, the muscle sustains some injury, as reflected in elevated creatine kinase levels. With appropriate thiamine supplementation, the muscle strength improves in 1 week, especially proximally, with the myalgia subsiding in 2 months and the creatine kinase level normal in 3 months.

Niacin deficiency

Niacin is the end product of tryptophan metabolism and is converted into nicotinamide adenine dinucleotide and nicotinamide adenine dinucleotide phosphate, coenzymes important in carbohydrate metabolism.

Pellagra, the classic niacin deficiency, is rare in developed countries, except if corn is the dietary staple, because corn lacks niacin and tryptophan. Foods rich in niacin include meat, fish, poultry, enriched grains and breads, and fortified cereals. The RDA (Recommended Daily Allowance) is 16 mg daily for men and 14 mg daily for women of niacin equivalent, with 1 mg niacin equivalent equal to 51 mg niacin or 60 mg tryptophan. It is not common in individuals who have alcoholism and malabsorption, because it is absorbed by simple diffusion with 30% of niacin protein bound [26]. A deficiency occurs in carcinoid syndrome, because tryptophan is converted to serotonin, not niacin. Biotransformation of tryptophan to nicotinic acid requires vitamins B2 and B6, iron, and copper, so one can also see secondary vitamin B6 deficiency. Pellagra affects the gastrointestinal tract, skin, and nervous system [27].

Patients have dermatitis, diarrhea, and dementia. The reddish-brown keratotic rash affects the face, chest, dorsum of the hands, and feet. There is anorexia, abdominal pain, diarrhea, and stomatitis. Neurologic problems are diffuse and complicated by other vitamin deficiencies. In fact, neuropathies may worsen if patients receive niacin supplementation without the rest of the vitamin B complex [28]. The peripheral neuropathy is indistinguishable from other causes, such as thiamine deficiency. There may be confusion with coma, spasticity, and myoclonus and progressive encephalopathy in alcoholic patients [27,29,30].

Laboratory studies include the urinary excretion of methylated metabolites, N-methylnicotinamide and its 2-pyridone derivative (N-methyl-2-pyridone-5-carboxamide) [27]. Treatment consists of oral nicotinic acid, 50 mg three times daily, or parenteral doses, 25 mg three times daily. Advanced pellagra is treated with intramuscular nicotinic acid, 50 to 100 mg three times daily for 3 to 4 days followed by oral supplementation [26]. In Parkinsonism, treatment with L-dopa, especially when given with a decarboxylase inhibitor (carbidopa) increases the risk for niacin deficiency. Supplementation with niacin may increase the efficacy of L-dopa by extending the length of time that L-dopa levels remain elevated in the brain [31]. Also, nicotinamide adenine dinucleotide (NADH), a coenzyme formed from niacin, is required for the synthesis of tetrahydrobiopterin, the cofactor for the enzyme (tyrosine hydroxylase) that catalyzes the conversion of tyrosine to L-dopa [32].

Riboflavin

The rare Strachan syndrome is partially related to a deficiency of this vitamin and causes orogenital dermatitis, painful sensory neuropathy, amblyopia, and deafness. It is found in severely malnourished populations and is believed to result from distal degeneration of central and peripheral processes of sensory neurons. Riboflavin supplementation seems to reverse the skin manifestations [33].

Vitamin B6

Vitamin B6 has three main active derivatives: pyridoxal, pyridoxine, and pyridoxamine [34]. Its cellular functions as a coenzyme in the form of pyridoxal phosphate (PLP) are important in metabolic reactions, involving amino acids, lipids, nucleic acid, and one carbon units, for gluconeogenesis, neurotransmitter, and hemoglobin biosynthesis [35]. The interconversion and metabolism depends on riboflavin, niacin, and zinc.

Niacin, carnitine, and folate also require vitamin B6 for their metabolism. Food sources are meat, fish, eggs, soybeans, nuts, and dairy products. It cannot be synthesized from exogenous sources and is absorbed by way of the intestine [35]. All forms are phosphorylated for metabolic trapping.

The RDA is 1.3 mg daily for men and 1.4 mg daily for women, with the upper limit (UL) being 100 mg daily. Administration of 2 mg of vitamin B6 daily after bariatric surgery has been shown to prevent deficiency [36,37]. Excess consumption in the range of 1 to 5 grams daily for 2 to 3 years can cause a pure sensory peripheral neuropathy [38,39], sensory ataxia, areflexia, impaired cutaneous and deep sensation, and a positive Romberg sign. These findings may reverse once excessive supplementation is withdrawn. A deficiency causes a microcytic hypochromic anemia, and treatment of 50 to 100 mg daily may prevent the development of neuropathy. Infants who have deficiencies may have seizures, but adults are more resistant.

Pregnant and lactating women, those taking estrogen, and the elderly are most at risk for a pyridoxine deficiency, which is more frequent with administration of vitamin B6 antagonists, isoniazid (INH), cycloserine, hydralazine, and penicillamine [40]. With INH one can get an associated neuropathy, including limb weakness and sensory ataxia [41]. It is dose related and associated with axonal degeneration and regeneration, affecting myelinated and unmyelinated fibers on sural biopsy [42]; it is reversible by discontinuing the drug or by supplementing the patient with vitamin B6 [43].

Treatment for Parkinsonism with L-dopa and a decarboxylase inhibitor may provoke a marginal vitamin B6 deficiency [44], which is important in Parkinson disease, because dopa decarboxylase catalyzes the conversion of dopa to dopamine and depends on pyridoxal phosphate, the activated form of vitamin B6. Some clinical trials of vitamin B6 supplementation to patients who have Parkinsonism suggest that tremor, muscle cramps, rigidity, bladder control, gait, and energy are improved, although further studies are needed to substantiate [45].

Vitamin B12

Cyanocobalamin (Cbl) is the chemical name for vitamin B12. The active forms are methyl Cbl and adenosyl Cbl [5]. Food sources are meat, eggs, and milk, and there are no adverse effects associated with excess Cbl intake. Vitamin B12 is essential in DNA synthesis, being a cofactor for folate-dependent methionine synthase, and mitochondrial-β-oxidation of fatty acids being a cofactor for methylmalonyl CoA mutase [34]. Stomach acid and pepsin dissociate Cbl from proteins and it binds with R protein secreted by the gastric of the small intestine, which is degraded in the neutral pH of the small intestine, and hydrolyzed by pancreatic enzymes to release the Cbl, which then binds with intrinsic factor (IF), secreted by gastric parietal cells. In the terminal ileum, the vitamin B12–IF complex finds an IF receptor and is absorbed by the intestinal mucosal cells. A deficiency of Cbl may cause pernicious anemia (PA), and one may also have an associated iron deficiency [5,46].

Neurologic manifestations of Cbl deficiency are caused by overproduction of myelinolytic tumor necrosis factor (TNF) alpha and reduced synthesis of epidermal growth factor and interleukin 6. Deficiencies are seen with metabolic problems and in the elderly. Those who develop MS before age 18 years also have lower serum vitamin B12 levels, suggesting that the deficiency may lead to vulnerability in the viral or immune mechanisms believed to cause MS, although MS may increase the need for vitamin B12 [47–49].

Causes of vitamin B12 deficiency are atrophic gastritis, achlorhydria-induced food Cbl malabsorption, acid reduction therapy with H2-blockers, ileal disease, resection with malabsorption, and, rarely, decreased dietary intake. Often the etiology is not known [50]. The neuropathy associated with vitamin B12 deficiency may be related to interference with methylation reactions in the CNS [51,52]. Myelopathy with and without neuropathy is seen with combined degeneration of the cervical and upper thoracic posterior columns [53,54]. In the white matter there are foci of myelin and axon destruction. MRI reveals signal change in the subcortical white matter and posterior and lateral columns [55,56], and electrodiagnosis reveals axonal degeneration with and without demyelination. There is sensorimotor axonopathy, possible multifocal alterations in conduction, abnormal somatosensory-evoked potentials in central sensory pathways, visual-evoked potentials, and motor-evoked potentials [56–59].

Cognitive impairment, optic neuropathy causing cacco-central scotoma, paresthesias, and polyneuropathy can coexist. The clinical picture most often consists of paresthesia starting in the lower extremities and spreading up to the trunk, difficulty walking, gait disturbance, and in advanced cases, sphincter dysfunction. The physical signs characteristically show spastic and ataxic gait with signs of peripheral neuropathy, ie, absent ankle reflexes. In some cases, Lhermitte sign may be observed. Cognitive impairment is not uncommon in this condition, and severity varies from mild irritability and mood disturbance to frank dementia [60]. Some patients may have high folate levels. The neurologic problems with low Cbl do not establish cause and effect of Cbl deficiency [61], which can also be seen with copper deficiency [62]. Laboratory findings include macrocytic red blood cells, megaloblastic anemia, and low serum Cbl [63,64]. Increased gastrin levels and markers for hypochlorhydria or achlorhydria are seen with pernicious anemia, and they have a high sensitivity and specificity for PA. These problems are also seen in 30% of elderly patients [58,65–67]. Clinically the patient may have glossitis, weight loss, and loss of appetite, and some patients may have orthostatic hypotension [7]. Diagnosis requires checking serum vitamin B12 level. A low level of vitamin B12 in serum in the setting of compatible clinical features, neuroimaging, and electrophysiologic studies establishes the diagnosis. In some cases of vitamin B12 deficiency, the vitamin B12 level could be within normal ranges. In such cases, serum methylmalonic acid and homocysteine, if elevated, help with the diagnosis [5]. Treatment with 3 to 5 μg daily may suffice if absorption is normal. Malabsorption secondary to achlorhydria may require parenteral supplementation with 50 to 100 µg daily [68]. Maintenance therapy is 1000 µg intramuscularly monthly [69]. Response of the hematologic derangement should be prompt and complete within 6 months. Alcohol abuse affects the enterohepatic recycling of Cbl, affecting folate metabolism, and accelerates the breakdown of folate. The anemia of Cbl deficiency may respond to folate therapy, but the response is often incomplete [70].

Folic acid

Folate or folic acid consists of pterin linked to p-aminobenzoic acid. It acts through its coenzyme by modifying, accepting, or transferring one-carbon moieties in single carbon reaction in metabolism of nucleic and amino acids. Biochemical pathways requiring folic acid include interconversion of serine and glycine, methionine cycle, histidine catabolism, thymidylate, and purine cycles. Methyl-tetrahydrofolate (methyl-THF) is the predominant folate [5]. Vitamin B12 acts as a coenzyme in the conversion of methyl-THF to THF, the biologically active form. Vitamin B12 deficiency can also cause folate deficiency [8,71,72] with the megaloblastic anemia being indistinguishable from Cbl deficiency [71].

Foods rich in folate include spinach, yeast, peanuts, liver, beans, and beer, with the bioavailability being 50% from food and 100% from folic monoglutamate. Fortification of grains and cereals has been mandated since 1998 in the United States for the prevention of neural tube defects, but folates in food are labile and are lost with boiling. The RDA is 400 µg daily of dietary folate equivalent, with the UL being 1000 µg daily. Absorption is in the proximal small intestines; cellular folate uptake occurs by passive diffusion, and folate undergoes polyglutamation that permits attachment to enzymes. Daily losses are 1% to 2% of body stores, and the body stores to daily requirement ratio is 100:1. Serum folate decreases within 3 weeks of decreased intake [73]. A deficiency can be seen within 3 months or faster in those who have low stores or alcoholism. Metabolism can be impaired by methotrexate or inborn errors of metabolism. Patients taking carbamazepine are susceptible to folate deficiency, because the drug impairs absorption [74]. Deficiency of folate is rarely seen in isolation except for small bowel disorders affecting absorption. These include inflammatory bowel disease, tropical sprue, or Celiac disease.

Alcoholic patients may have a deficiency of folic acid, usually in combination with other vitamins.

Neurologic problems are less common than they are with other nutrient deficiencies. Myeloneuropathy or polyneuropathy, including retrobulbar optic neuropathy, can be seen in association with folate deficiency or can be associated with affective psychiatric disorders [75,76].

Treatment of folate deficiency is 1 mg folate three times daily, followed by 1 mg daily. Parenteral administration of 1 to 5 mg daily is appropriate for more ill patients. Women who have epilepsy should take 0.4 mg for prophylaxis against neural tube defects.

Vitamin D

Vitamin D has several active metabolites, with 25-hydroxyvitamin D levels less than 50 nmol/L in the serum being associated with increased body sway and decreased neuromuscular coordination, whereas a level less than 30 nmol/L is associated with decreased muscle strength. There is an osteomalacic myopathy that causes one to have difficulty getting up from a chair, an inability to ascend stairs, and diffuse muscle pain. It is difficult to quantitate this loss of strength, given its predilection for proximal muscles, although electrodiagnosis can confirm a myopathic pattern with decreased motor unit amplitude and duration and increased polyphasicity [77]. A subclinical neuropathy can cause decreased nerve conduction velocities of the ulnar and peroneal nerves [78].

The skin can produce 80% to 90% of necessary vitamin D after exposure to UVB radiation, with hypovitaminosis D being more common in elderly individuals living in northern latitudes [79]. The extent to which one's body is covered with clothing or even sunscreen also affects the skin's ability to synthesize vitamin D. Hypovitaminosis D-related myopathy has been diagnosed in immigrant teenagers who were veiled [80].

Vitamin D must undergo two hydroxylations in the liver and kidney to become the biologically active form, $1,25(OH)_2D$, with the conversion in the kidney regulated by parathyroid hormone. Other regulators include calcium, phosphate, growth hormone, and prolactin [77]. A vitamin D binding protein (DBP) is a mediator of the effects of 25 OHD in muscle, and this active form, 25 OHD, may have more effect on striated skeletal muscle.

Calcium works together with vitamin D to maintain bone health in the human body [81,82]. Vitamin D works through its active form, $1,25(OH)_2D$. The primary action of $1,25(OH)_2D$ is to promote intestinal absorption of calcium and phosphorus through the small intestine. This reaction is regulated by parathyroid hormone. Moreover, calcium is important in nerve and muscle functions [83]. Calcium is mainly absorbed in the duodenum and proximal jejunum, whereas vitamin D is absorbed mainly in the jejunum and ileum [84]. In Roux-en-Y gastric bypass and biliopancreatic diversion, calcium and vitamin D deficiency predictably occur. Possible causes include bypassing the duodenum and proximal jejunum, food intolerance, and fat malabsorption. The frequencies of calcium and vitamin D deficiencies were reportedly 10% and 50%, respectively, after RYGB [85]. The deficiency results in osteoporosis and osteomalacia. In one study, 800 IU of cholecalciferol in combination with 1200 mg of elemental calcium reduced hip fractures and other non-vertebral fractures after 18 months of treatment [86]. There is a strong interdependency of the vitamin D deficiency with low levels of serum Ca and high levels of parathyroid hormone, so all three of these need to be evaluated. Increased secretion of parathyroid hormone, induced by vitamin D deficiency, contributes to bone fragility through loss of bone matrix and minerals, with decreased bone density at the hip and increased bone turnover [87].

Severe vitamin D deficiency in children causes rickets. At older ages, there is predominantly a myopathy (osteomalacia myopathy) affecting proximal strength, which may cause prominent muscle pain. A patient typically presents with progressive proximal weakness involving predominantly lower limbs, with gait difficulty, waddling gait, and difficulty rising from a chair or going up stairs. Physical examination reveals proximal weakness in the upper limbs and the muscles of the trunk [88,89]. There is conflicting information about the findings on electrodiagnosis. Although the myopathy can be detected, other investigators have suggested slowing in the nerve conduction studies. Muscle biopsies have confirmed more atrophy of type II muscle fibers, which are fast and strong and recruited first to avoid falling. Because these fibers are preferentially affected in vitamin D deficiency, it may explain the high fall risk in vitamin D-deficient elderly patients [77].

Measurement of serum vitamin D, urine calcium, serum bone alkaline phosphatase (BAP), and serum parathyroid hormone (PTH) levels would help establish the diagnosis. In general, serum vitamin D and 24-hour urine calcium are decreased (total 25 OHD < 15 ng/mL), and the levels of BAP and PTH are elevated [90]. Treatment with vitamin D supplement results in definite improvement in strength and pain [88,91]. If patients are deficient in vitamin D and calcium, the recommended supplements are 800 IU of cholecalciferol in combination with 1200 mg of elemental calcium [77]. After bariatric surgery, the recommended vitamin D supplementation is 50,000 IU of vitamin D3 (cholecalciferol) or vitamin D2 (ergocalciferol) once per week [90]. There is some evidence that vitamin D deficiency may be associated with an increased risk for type I diabetes, multiple sclerosis, rheumatoid arthritis, hypertension, cardiovascular heart disease, and cancers. Some suggest that yearly measurements of 25-hydroxyvitamin D should be part of the annual physical examination [81].

There is some evidence that the prevalence of MS is highest in regions where the vitamin D supplies are lowest and there is less environmental exposure to the sun, which limits vitamin D synthesis. Administration of one of the active metabolites of vitamin D, $1,25\text{-}OD_2D$, reduced disease activity in mice and rats with experimental allergic encephalomyelitis, suggesting some immune-mediated suppression of disease.

Supplementation with vitamin D for patients who have MS may therefore help to suppress the immunologic aspects of the disease and decrease bone resorption, fractures, and muscle weakness [77]. An associated decrease in calcium can cause a change in solubilized proteins from mouse brain tissue to cause abnormalities similar to MS plaque [47].

Vitamin E

Alpha tocopherol is the active form of vitamin E, which typically includes supplements containing esters that prolong the shelf life, preventing oxidation [92]. Foods containing vitamin E include vegetable oils, leafy vegetables, fruits, meat, nuts, and unprocessed cereal grains. Bioavailability depends on the food fat content and is better from enriched cereals than supplements [93]. RDA is 15 mg daily, with the UL being 1000 mg daily.

Alpha tocopherol is an antioxidant and free radical scavenger that protects the cellular membrane from oxidative stress and inhibits the peroxidation of polyunsaturated fatty acids of membrane phospholipids. Absorption efficiency is less than 50% and requires bile acids, fatty acids, and monoglycerides for micelle formation. Biliary and pancreatic secretions are required for absorption. It takes 2 years for adipose tissue levels to reach steady state with dietary intake changes [94].

A deficiency is never caused by a dietary insufficiency, but rather is associated with Crohn disease, celiac disease, cystic fibrosis, blind loop syndrome, or small bowel resection. Another problem may result from inadequate intake with parenteral nutrition to maintain stores [95].

There is some suggestion that later development of Parkinson disease is associated with a low intake of vitamin E-rich food earlier in life [96]. Neurologically, deficiency causes a spinocerebellar syndrome with variable peripheral nerve involvement [97–99]. One may see ataxia, hyporeflexia, proprioceptive, or vibratory loss. Cutaneous sensations are affected less. There may be dysarthria, tremor, nystagmus, ophthalmoplegia, ptosis, pigmentary retinopathy, or myopathy, which is rare in humans [100,101].

Biopsies from the sural nerve reveal centrally-directed fibers of large myelinated neurons most involved [102].

Levels of vitamin E depend on serum lipids, cholesterol, and very low density, with hyperlipids increasing vitamin E. With a deficiency, serum vitamin E levels may not be detectable, but fat malabsorption with increased stool fat and decreased serum carotene levels may be present. Treatment when the deficiency is associated with malabsorption is 200 IU per kg daily of intramuscular di-x tocopherol (0.8–2.0 IU/kg/day) [103]. With cholestatic liver disease, treatment with fat-soluble vitamin E is ineffective because of fat malabsorption. A water-soluble product helps increase levels of vitamin E in this case.

Copper

Copper deficiency in animal species does cause a myelopathy. Ruminants develop swayback. In humans, Menkes disease occurs, which is caused by a congenital deficiency [104]. Myelopathy or myeloneuropathy may resemble a vitamin B12 deficiency [105,106]. Copper and cyanocobalamin deficiencies may coexist, so if one still has neurologic problems after vitamin B12 supplementation, copper deficiency should be considered.

Copper functions as a prosthetic group in metalloenzymes, which act as oxidases that transfer electrons in mitochondria and help maintain the structure and function of the nervous system [105,107,108]. It also plays an important role in iron metabolism, the neurotransmitter system (dopamine β-hydroxylase), and collagen synthesis (lysyl oxidase).

The RDA for copper is 900 μg daily, with the UL being 10,000 μg daily. Foods rich in copper are organ meats, seafood, nuts, seeds, wheat bran cereals, whole grain products, and cocoa products. Tea, potatoes, milk, and chicken do not contain much copper. Deficiency can be seen with prolonged parenteral nutrition use [109].

Absorption is by saturable active transport at lower levels of intake and passive diffusion at higher levels of intake in the stomach and throughout the small intestine. It is bound to albumin and transported by way of the portal vein to the liver for uptake there. Parenchymal cells then released into plasma are bound to ceruloplasmin 95% of the time. Urinary excretion is low, and excretion of copper into the gastrointestinal tract is the major pathway regulating copper homeostasis, preventing deficiency. Copper absorption can be inhibited by high zinc intake because of a zinc-induced high level of metallothionein. Metallothionein has a high affinity for copper, and the copper-bound metallothionein is sloughed off into the intestine, thus losing copper from the body. High zinc intake can precipitate copper deficiency in a predisposed patient [110]. Copper absorption into intestinal mucosa requires copper transporters (Ctr1 copper transporter and DCT-1) [111]. It is then transported to ATP7A to be exported from the intestinal cells into the circulation. Dietary factors affecting bioavailability are acid, amount of copper, molybdenum, or zinc intake, which, when excessive, reduces copper absorption and may possibly compete for common transport. Problems are usually related to impaired absorption, such as following bariatric surgery [5], with acquired deficiency being rare because of the ubiquitous distribution.

Neurologic manifestations include myelopathy with a spastic gait and sensory ataxia secondary to sensory loss from dorsal column involvement [112,113], similar to a vitamin B12 deficiency. There can be CNS demyelination and optic neuritis [114]. Neurogenic bladder symptoms and Lhermitte signs may be observed. Brisk knee reflexes, extensor plantar response, and absent ankle reflexes are common physical signs. Electrodiagnosis reveals a peripheral neuropathy, sensorimotor axonal type; somatosensory-evoked potentials are consistent with a central delay; visual-evoked potentials are prolonged. Spinal MRI may have an increased signal on T2-weighted images in the paramedian cervical and thoracic cord [113]. Hematologically there may be an anemia, neutropenia of unclear etiology, left shift granulocytosis with ringed sideroblasts but not sideroblastic anemia, or there may be no hematologic problems [5]. In second generation rats, copper deficiency produces low dopamine levels in the corpus striatum and results in clinical signs similar to Parkinson disease [115], although in humans there is no evidence that copper supplementation is efficacious for the treatment of Parkinsonism. In animal studies, copper deficiency causes defective myelination [116]. Serum copper is not totally adequate to assess copper stores [117]. Ceruloplasmin is an acute phase reactant, and its increase parallels the increase in copper levels. It is seen during pregnancy, in liver disease, malignancy, hematologic disease, myocardial infarction, smoking, diabetes mellitus, uremia, and inflammatory and infectious diseases.

Treatment of low serum copper levels and low ceruloplasmin levels is copper supplementation orally, 2 mg daily. Response is fast, and one can reassess serum copper to determine the adequacy of replacement and reassess hematologic and sensory symptoms [118], with hematologic improvement being more dramatic than neurologic improvement. Neuroimaging studies may normalize after treatment [112]. The frequency of copper deficiency after bariatric surgery is covered elsewhere in this issue.

Zinc

Zinc metabolism can be altered in diseases like Parkinsonism, in which there is oxidative stress [119]. In guinea pigs that were zinc deficient, motor nerve conduction velocities were decreased and there was abnormal locomotion and posture [52]. Catabolic states associated with inflammation or trauma may increase the use of zinc and may lead to a relative deficiency.

As mentioned, zinc can also induce copper deficiency, with treatment being discontinuing zinc, but hyperzincemia can accompany copper deficiency without exogenous zinc supplementation. Zinc levels therefore should also be checked in copper deficiency, as noted [120].

Summary

The effects of multiple nutritional deficiencies on neuromuscular problems have been postulated for many years, and other relationships are suspected. There is more literature documenting nutritional deficiencies in the elderly, chronically ill (children and adults), and those who do not take in adequate nutrients or calories because their energy intake is in the form of alcohol or because they are anorexic. As individuals lose weight from chronic disease or the ravages of alcoholism, anorexia, or failure to thrive, they may develop other neurologic problems, such as entrapment neuropathies from mechanical pressure on vulnerable peripheral nerves. These may include the ulnar nerve at the elbow and the peroneal nerve at the fibular head, with malnutrition possibly predisposing the nerves to more damage from direct pressure.

It is difficult to study some of the causative factors, because these individuals may have multiorgan failure, which affects absorption, and they may take vitamin supplements that are not reported on their health history. In fact, as discussed, excessive consumption of some nutrients may also have deleterious effects on one's health, and key nutrients may be lacking with metabolic disease, prolonged parenteral nutrition, or secondary to a medication. One's suboptimal diet may not be considered when evaluating specific diseases, plus some individuals on parenteral or enteral nutrition may be taking additional calories and nutrients orally, with the combination being insufficient to meet their requirements. Supplementation may need to include more than one nutrient. It is helpful to treat vitamin B deficiencies with the entire B complex, to provide calcium with vitamin D, and to always ensure adequate calories so there is sufficient energy, to maintain protein stores, and to consume key nutrients. These inter-relationships may not be recognized by patients and their health care providers, and patients who rely on supplements rather than a balanced diet may not ingest the ideal proportion of different nutrients. The focus here has been on what is known about the relationship between key nutrients and neuromuscular disease, and this article supports obtaining a detailed nutrition assessment in at-risk patients. Much remains to be studied. There are few data that define the beneficial effect of a nutritional supplement on the course of a particular disease, yet commercialism and diet fads proliferate. Many individuals spend their limited financial resources on supplements rather than nutritious food. With more nutrition education regarding food labeling, research, and attention to the critical role that nutrition plays in one's health, some of these secondary effects of nutritional deficiencies may be lessened or reversed, enhancing one's sense of well being as one ages or lives with a chronic illness.

References

[1] Williams FH, Hopkins B. Nutrition management in rehabilitation patients. General rehabilitation text. Delisa FA, Gans BM, editors. 2004; 4th edition. p. 1267–87.
[2] Shlomo Y, Smith GD, Marmot MG, et al. Dietary fat in the epidemiology of multiple sclerosis: has the situation been adequately addressed? Neuroepidemiology 1992;11(4–6):214–25.
[3] Tola MR, Granieri S, Malagu L, et al. Dietary habits and multiple sclerosis. A retrospective study in Ferrara, Italy. Acta Neurol (Napoli) 1994;16(4):189–97.
[4] Butterworth RF, Herous M. Effect of pyrithiamine treatment and subsequent thiamine rehabilitation on regional cerebral amino acids and thiamine-dependent enzymes. J Neurochem 1989;52:1079–84.
[5] Kumar N. Nutritional neuropathies. Neurol Clin 2007;25:209–55.
[6] McCormick D. Niacin, riboflavin and thiamin. In: Stipanuk M, editor. Biochemical, physiological, molecular aspects of human nutrition. St. Louis (MO): Saunders Elsevier; 2006. p. 665–92.
[7] Phuapradit P. Vitamin deficiencies, intoxications and gastrointestinal disorders. In: Swash M, Oxbury J, editors. Clinical neurology. New York: Churchill Livingstone; 1991. p. 1695–710.
[8] Ukleja A, Stone R. Medical and gastroenterologic management of the post-bariatric surgery patient. J Clin Gastroenterol 2004;38:312–21.
[9] Ohnishi A, Tsuji S, Igisu H, et al. Beriberi neuropathy. Morphometric study of sural nerve. J Neurol Sci 1980;45:177–90.
[10] Metz J. Cobalamin deficiency and the pathogenesis of nervous system disease. Annu Rev Nutr 1992;12:59–79.
[11] Koike H, Misu K, Hattori N, et al. Postgastrectomy polyneuropathy with thiamine deficiency. J Neurol Neurosurg Psychiatry 2001;71:357–62.
[12] Hornabrook RW. Alcoholic neuropathy. Am J Clin Nutr 1961;9:398–403.
[13] Butterworth RF. Thiamin. In: Shils ME, Shike M, Ross AC, editors. Modern nutrition in health and disease. 10th edition. Baltimore (MD): Lippincott Williams and Wilkins; 2006. p. 426–33.

[14] So YT, Simon RP. Deficiency diseases of the nervous system. In: Bradley WG, Daroff RB, Fenichel GM, et al, editors. Neurology in clinical practice, vol. II. 4th editionPhiladelphia: Butterworth Heinemann; 2004. p. 1693–708.

[15] Caine D, Halliday GM, Kril JJ, et al. Operational criteria for the classification of chronic alcoholics: identification of Wernicke's encephalopathy. J Neurol Neurosurg Psychiatry 1997;62:51–60.

[16] Dohery MJ, Watson NF, Uchino K, et al. Diffusion abnormalities on patients with Wernicke encephalopathy. Neurology 2002;58:655–7.

[17] Harper C. Wernicke's encephalopathy: a more common disease than realized. A neuropathological study of 51 cases. J Neurol Neurosurg Psychiatry 1979;42:226–31.

[18] Singh S, Kumar A. Wernicke encephalopathy after obesity surgery. Neurology 2007;68:1–5.

[19] Shaw S, Lieber CS. Alcoholism. In: Nutritional support of medical practice. Schneider, et al, editors. 2nd edition. Harper & Row Publishers; Philadelphia;1983. p. 236–9.

[20] Dreyfus PM. Thiamine and the nervous system: an overview. J Nutr Sci Vitaminol (Tokoyo) 1967;22(Suppl):13–6.

[21] Talwar D, Davidson H, Cooney J, et al. Vitamin B(1) status assessed by direct measurement of thiamin pyrophosphate in erythrocytes or whole blood by HPLC: comparison with erythrocyte transketolase activation assay. Clin Chem 2000;46:704–10.

[22] Roman GC. Nutritional disorders of the nervous system. In: Shils ME, Shike M, Ross AC, editors. Modern nutrition in health and disease. 10th edition. Baltimore (MD): Lippincott Williams and Wilkins; 2006. p. 1362–80.

[23] Woelk H, Lethrl S, Bitsch R, et al. Benfotiamine in treatment of alcoholic polyneuropathy: an 8 week randomized controlled study (BAP I study). Alcohol Alcohol 1998;33:631–8.

[24] Salas-Salvado J, Garcia-Lorda P, Cuatrecasas G, et al. Wernicke's syndrome after bariatric surgery. Clin Nutr 2000;19:371–3.

[25] Koike H, Watanabe H, Inukai A, et al. Myopathy in thiamine deficiency: analysis of a case. J Neurol Sci 2006;249:175–9.

[26] Bourgeois C, Cervantes-Laurean D, Moss J. Niacin. In: Shile ME, Shike M, Ross AC, editors. Modern nutrition in health and disease. 10th edition. Baltimore (MD): Lippincott Williams and Wilkins; 2006. p. 442–51.

[27] Institute of Medicine. Niacin. In: Food and Nutrition Board, editor. Dietary reference intakes: thiamin, riboflavin, niacin, vitamin B6, folate, vitamin B12, pantothenic acid, biotin, and choline. Washington, DC: National Academy Press; 1998. p. 123–49.

[28] Wadia NH, Swami RK. Pattern of nutritional deficiency disorders of nervous system in Bombay. Neurol India 1970;18:207.

[29] Spies TD, Aring CD. The effect of vitamin B1 on the peripheral neuritis of pellagra. JAMA 1938;110:1081–4.

[30] Spies TD, Vilter RW, Ashe WF. Pellagra, beriberi and riboflavin deficiency in human beings: diagnosis and treatment. JAMA 1939;113:931–7.

[31] Black MJ, Brandt RB. Nicotinic acid or N-methyl nicotinamide prolongs elevated brain dopa and dopamine in L-dopa treatment. Biochem Med Metab Biol 1986;36(2):244–51.

[32] Vrecko K, Birkmayer JGD, Krainz J, et al. Stimulation of dopamine biosynthesis in cultured PC 12 phaeochromocytoma cells by the coenzyme nicotinamide adeninedinucleotide (NADH). J Neural Transm Park Dis Dement Sect 1993;5(2):147–56.

[33] McCormick DB. Riboflavin. In: Shils ME, Shike M, Ross AC, editors. Modern nutrition in health and disease. 10th edition. Baltimore (MD): Lippincott Williams and Wilkins; 2006. p. 434–41.

[34] Shane B. Folic acid, vitamin B12, and vitamin B6. In: Stipanuk M, editor. Biochemical, physiological, molecular aspects of human nutrition. St. Louis (MO): Saunders Elsevier; 2006. p. 693–732.

[35] Mackey AD, Davis SR, Gregory JFI. Vitamin B6. In: Shils ME, Shike M, Ross AC, et al, editors. Modern nutrition health and disease. 10th edition. Baltimore (MD): Lippincott Williams and Wilkins; 2006. p. 452–61.

[36] Turkki P, Ingerman L, Schroeder L, et al. Plasma pyridoxal phosphate as indicator of vitamin B6 status in morbidly obese women after gastric restriction surgery. Nutrition 1989;5(4):229–35.

[37] Provenzale D, Reinhold R, Golner B, et al. Evidence for diminished B12 absorption after gastric bypass: oral supplementation does not prevent low plasma B12 levels in bypass patients. J Am Coll Nutr 1992;11(1):29–35.

[38] Schaumburg H, Kaplan J, Windebank A, et al. Sensory neuropathy from pyridoxine abuse. A new megavitamin syndrome. N Engl J Med 1983;309:445–8.

[39] Parry GJ, Bredesen DE. Sensory neuropathy with low-dose pyridoxine. Neurology 1985; 35:1466–8.

[40] Bhagavan HN, Brin M. Drug-vitamin B6 interaction. Curr Concepts Nutr 1983;12:1–12.

[41] Goldman AL, Braman SS. Isoniazid: a review with emphasis on adverse effects. Chest 1972; 62:71–7.

[42] Ochoa J. Isoniazid neuropathy in man: quantitative electron microscopic study. Brain 1970; 93:831–50.

[43] Victor M, Adams RD. The neuropathology of experimental vitamin B6 deficiency in monkeys. Am J Clin Nutr 1956;4:346–53.

[44] Frank O, Jaslow SP, Thind I, et al. Superiority of periodic intramuscular vitamins over daily oral vitamins in maintaining normal vitamin titers in a geriatric population. Am J Clin Nutr 1977;30:630.

[45] Vainshtok AV. Treatment of Parkinsonism with large doses of vitamin B6. Sov Med 1979;7: 14–9.

[46] Carmel R, Weiner JM, Johnson CS. Iron deficiency occurs frequently in patients with pernicious anemia. JAMA 1987;257:1081–3.

[47] Werbach MR, Moss J. Textbook of nutritional medicine, multiple sclerosis. California: 3rd line press; 1999. p. 531–41.

[48] Carmel R. Cobalamin (vitamin B12). In: Shils ME, Shike M, Ross AC, et al, editors. Modern nutrition in health and disease. 10th edition. Baltimore (MD): Lippincott Williams and Wilkins; 2006. p. 482–97.

[49] Lindenbaum J, Healton EB, Savage DG, et al. Neuropsychiatric disorders caused by cobalamin deficiency in the absence of anemia or macrocytosis. N Engl J Med 1988;318: 1720–8.

[50] Marcuard SP, Albernaz L, Khazanie PG. Omeprazole therapy causes of cyanocobalamin (vitamin B12). Ann Intern Med 1994;120:211–5.

[51] Weir DG, Scott JM. The biochemical basis of the neuropathy in cobalamin deficiency. Baillieres Clin Haematol 1995;8(3):479–97.

[52] Werbach MR, Moss J. Textbook of nutritional medicine, neuralgia and neuropathy. California: 3rd line press; 1999. p. 552–7.

[53] Russell JSR, Batten FE, Collier J. Subacute combined degeneration of the spinal cord. Brain 1900;23:39–110.

[54] Pant SS, Asbury AK, Richardson EP Jr. The myelopathy of pernicious anemia. A neuropathological reappraisal. Acta Neurol Scand 1968;44(Suppl 5)1:1–36.

[55] Timms SR, Cure JK, Kurent JE. Subacute combined degeneration of the spinal cord: MR findings. AJNR Am J Neuroradiol 1993;14:1224–7.

[56] Hemmer B, Glocker FX, Schumacher M, et al. Subacute combined degeneration: clinical, electrophysiological, and magnetic resonance imaging findings. J Neurol Neurosurg Psychiatry 1998;65:822–7, 1618–22.

[57] Fine EJ, Hallet M. Neurophysiological study of subacute combined degeneration. J Neurol Sci 1980;45:331–6.

[58] McCombe PA, McLeod JG. The peripheral neuropathy of vitamin B12 deficiency. J Neurol Sci 1984;66:117–26.

[59] Heyer EJ, Simpson DM, Bodis-Wollner I, et al. Nitrous oxide: clinical and electrophysiologic investigation of neurologic complications. Neurology 1986;36:1618–22.

[60] Healton EB, Savage DG, Brust JC, et al. Neurologic aspects of cobalamin deficiency. Medicine (Baltimore) 1991;70:229–45.

[61] Carmel R, Green R, Rosenblatt DS, et al. Update on cobalamin, folate, and homocysteine. Hematology 2003;1:62–81.

[62] Carmel R, Melnyk S, James SJ. Cobalamin deficiency with and without neurologic abnormalities: differences in homocysteine and methionine metabolism. Blood 2003;101:3302–8.

[63] Green R, Kinsella LJ. Current concepts in the diagnosis of cobalamin deficiency. Neurology 1995;45:1435–40.

[64] Snow CF. Laboratory diagnosis of vitamin B12 and folate deficiency: a guide for the primary care physician. Arch Intern Med 1999;159:1289–98.

[65] Hurwitz A, Brady DA, Schaal SE, et al. Gastric acidity in older adults. JAMA 1997;278: 659–62.

[66] White WB, Reik L Jr, Cutlip DE. Pernicious anemia seen initially as orthostatic hypotension. Arch Intern Med 1981;141:1543–4.

[67] Eisenhofer G, Lambie DG, Johnson RH, et al. Deficient catecholamine release as the basis of orthostatic hypotension in pernicious anemia. J Neurol Neurosurg Psychiatry 1982;45: 1053–5.

[68] Verhaeverbeke I, Mets T, Mulkens K, et al. Normalization of low vitamin B12 serum levels in older people by oral treatment. J Am Geriatr Soc 1997;45:124–5.

[69] Lederle FA. Oral cobalamin for pernicious anemia. Medicine's best kept secret? JAMA 1991;265:94–5.

[70] Halsted CH. Folate deficiency in alcoholism. Am J Clin Nutr 1980;33:2736–40.

[71] Institute of Medicine. Folate. In: Food and Nutrition Board, editor. Dietary reference intakes for thioamine, riboflavin, niacin, vitamin B6, folate, vitamin B12, pantothenic acid, biotin, and choline. Washington, DC: National Academy Press, National Academy of Sciences; 1998. p. 196–305.

[72] Carmel R. Folic acid. In: Shils ME, Shike M, Ross AC, et al, editors. Modern nutrition in health and disease. 10th edition. Baltimore (MD): Lippincott Williams and Wilkins; 2006. p. 470–81.

[73] Eichner ER, Pierce HI, Hillman RS. Folate balance in dietary-induced megaloblastic anemia. N Engl J Med 1971;284:933–8.

[74] Hendel J, Mogens D, Lennart G, et al. The effects of carbamazepine and valproate on folate metabolism. Acta Neurol Scand 1984;69(4):226–31.

[75] Shorvon SD, Carney MW, Chanarin I, et al. The neuropsychiatry of megaloblastic anemia. BMJ 1980;281:1036–8.

[76] Lopez-Hernan. Peripheral and optic. Rev Neurol 2003;37:Oct. p. 20.

[77] Pfeifer M, Begerow B, Minne HW. Vitamin D and muscle function. Osteoporos Int 2002; 13:187–94.

[78] Skaria J, Katiyar BC, Nrivastava TP, et al. Myopathy and neuropathy associated with osteomalacia. Acta Neurol Scand 1975;51(1):37–58.

[79] Webb AR, Pilbeam C, Hanafin N, et al. An evaluation of the relative contributions of exposure to sunlight and of diet to the circulating concentrations of 25 hydroxyvitamin D in an elderly nursing home population in Boston. Am J Clin Nutr 1990;51:1075–81.

[80] Vander Heyden JJC, Verrips A, ter Laak HJ, et al. Hypovitaminosis D related myopathy in immigrant teenagers. Neuropediatrics 2004;35:290–2.

[81] Holick J. Vitamin D. In: Stipanuk M, editor. Biochemical, physiological, molecular aspects of human nutrition. St. Louis (MO): Saunders Elsevier; 2006. p. 863–83.

[82] Wood R. Calcium and phosphorus. In: Stipanuk M, editor. Biochemical, physiological, molecular aspects of human nutrition. St. Louis (MO): Saunders Elsevier; 2006. p. 863–83.

[83] Malinowski S. Nutritional and metabolic complications of bariatric surgery. Am J Med Sci 2006;331(4):219–25.

[84] Alvarez-Leite J. Nutritional deficiency secondary to bariatric surgery. Curr Opin Clin Nutr Metab Care 2004;7:569–75.

[85] Shah M, Simha V, Garg A. Review: long term impact of bariatric surgery on body weight, comorbidities, and nutritional status. J Clin Endocrinol Metab 2006;91:4223–31.

[86] Chapuy MC, Arlot ME, Duboeuf F, et al. Vitamin D3 and calcium to prevent hip fractures in elderly women. N Engl J Med 1992;327:1637–42.

[87] Ooms ME, Roos JC, Bezemer PD, et al. Prevention of bone loss by vitamin D supplementation in elderly women: a randomized double-blind trial. J clin Endocrinol Metab 1995;80:1052–8.

[88] Russell J. Osteomalacic myopathy. Muscle Nerve 1994;17:578–80.

[89] Reginato A, Falasca G, Pappu R, et al. Musculoskeletal manifestations of osteomalacia: report of 26 cases and literature review. Semin Arthritis Rheum 1999;28(5):287–304.

[90] McMahon M, Sarr M, Clark M, et al. Clinical management after bariatric surgery: value of a multidisciplinary approach. Mayo Clin Proc 2006;81(Suppl 10):S34–45.

[91] Smith R, Stern G. Myopathy, osteomalacia and hyperparathyroidism. Brain 1967;90(3): 593–602.

[92] Cheeseman KH, Holley AE, Kelly FJ, et al. Biokinetics in humans of RRR-alpha-tocopherol: the free phenol, acetate ester, and succinate ester forms of vitamin E. Free Radic Biol Med 1995;19:591–8.

[93] Hayes K, Pronczuk A, Perlman D. Vitamin E in fortified cow milk uniquely enriches human plasma lipoproteins. Am J Clin Nutr 2001;74:211–8.

[94] Hendelman GJ, Epstein WL, Peerson J, et al. Human adipose alpha-tocopherol and gamma-tocopherol kinetics during and after 1 year of alpha-tocopherol supplementation. Am J Clin Nutr 1994;59:1025–32.

[95] Steephen AC, Traber MJ, Ito Y, et al. Vitamin E status of patients receiving long-term parenteral nutrition: is vitamin E supplementation adequate? JPEN J Parenter Enteral Nutr 1991;15:647–52.

[96] Golbe L, Farrell TM, Davis PH, et al. Followup study of early life protective and risk factors in Parkinson's disease. Mov Disord 1990;5(1):66–70.

[97] Harding AE. Vitamin E and the nervous system. Crit Rev Neurobiol 1987;3:89–103.

[98] Sokol RJ. Vitamin E deficiency and neurologic disease. Annu Rev Nutr 1988;8:351–73.

[99] Ben Hamida M, Belal S, Sirugo G, et al. Friedreich's ataxia phenotype not linked to chromosome 9 and associated with selective autosomal recessive vitamin E deficiency in two Tunisian families. Neurology 1993;43:2179–83.

[100] Tomasi LG. Reversibility of human myopathy caused by vitamin E deficiency. Neurology 1979;29:1182–6.

[101] Burck U, Goebel HH, Kuhlenahl HD, et al. Neuromyopathy and vitamin E deficiency in man. Neuropediatrics 1981;12:267–78.

[102] Sokol RJ, Bove KE, Heubi JE, et al. Vitamin E deficiency during chronic childhood cholestasis: presence of sural nerve lesion prior to $2\frac{1}{2}$ years of age. J Pediatr 1983;103:197–204.

[103] Sokol RJ, Guggenheim MA, Iannaccone ST, et al. Improved neurologic function after long-term correction of vitamin E deficiency in children with chronic cholestasis. N Engl J Med 1985;313:1580–6.

[104] Tan N, Urich H. Menkes' disease and swayback. A comparative study of two copper deficiency syndromes. J Neurol Sci 1983;62:95–113.

[105] Kumar N, Gross JB Jr, Ahlskog JE. Copper deficiency myelopathy produces a clinical picture like subacute combined degeneration. Neurology 2004;63:33–9.

[106] Kumar N. Copper deficiency myelopathy (human swayback). Mayo Clin Proc 2006;81(10): 1371–84.

[107] Institute of Medicine. Copper. In: Food and Nutrition Board, editor. Dietary reference intakes for vitamin A, vitamin K, arsenic, boron, chromium, copper, iodine, iron, manganese, molybdenum, nickel, silicon, vanadium, and zinc. Washington DC: National Academy Press; 2000. p. 224–57.

[108] Turnlund JR. Copper. In: Shils ME, Shike M, Ross AC, et al, editors. Modern nutrition in health and disease. 10th edition. Baltimore (MD): Lippincott Williams and Wilkins; 2006. p. 286.

[109] Karpel JT, Peden VH. Copper deficiency in long-term parenteral nutrition. J Pediatr 1972; 80:32–6.

[110] Kumar N, Crum B, Petersen R, et al. Copper deficiency myelopathy. Arch Neurol 2004;61: 762–6.

[111] Grider A. Zinc, copper and manganese. In: Stipanuk M, editor. Biochemical, physiological, molecular aspects of human nutrition. St. Louis (MO): Saunders Elsevier; 2006. p. 1043–67.

[112] Kumar N, McEvoy K, Ahlskog E. Myelopathy due to copper deficiency following gastro-intestinal surgery. Arch neurol 2003;60:1782–5.

[113] Kumar N, Ahlskog J, Klein C, et al. Imaging features of copper deficiency myelopathy: a study of 25 cases. Neuroradiology 2006;48(2):78–83.

[114] Gregg XT, Redy V, Prchal JT. Copper deficiency masquerading as myelodysplastic syndrome. Blood 2002;100:1493–5.

[115] Werbach MR, Moss J. Textbook of nutritional medicine, Parkinson's disease. California: 3rd line press; 1999. p. 604–15.

[116] Underwood EJ. Trace elements in human and animal nutrition. 4th edition. New York: Academic Press; 1971.

[117] Uauy R, Castillo-Duran C, Fisberg J, et al. Red cell superoxide dismutase activity as an index of human copper nutrition. J Nutr 1985;115:1650–5.

[118] Danks DM. Copper deficiency in humans. Annu Rev Nutr 1988;8:235–57.

[119] Cuajungao MP, Lees GJ. Zinc metabolism in the brain: relevance to human neurodegenerative disorders. Neurobiol Dis 1997;4(3–4):137–69.

[120] Kumar N, Elliott MF, Hoyer JD, et al. Myelodysplasia myeloneuropathy and copper deficiency. Mayo Clin Proc 2005;80:943–6.

ELSEVIER
SAUNDERS

Phys Med Rehabil Clin N Am
19 (2008) 149–162

PHYSICAL MEDICINE
AND REHABILITATION
CLINICS OF
NORTH AMERICA

Peripheral Neuropathy in Pregnancy

E. Wayne Massey, MD[a], Kathryn A. Stolp, MD[b],*

[a]Department of Neurology, Duke University Medical Center, Box 3909,
Durham, NC 27710, USA
[b]Mayo Clinic College of Medicine, Department of Physical Medicine and Rehabilitation,
Mayo Clinic Rochester, 200 1st Street SW, Rochester, MN 55905, USA

Peripheral neuropathy, mononeuropathy and polyneuropathy, are not common in pregnancy. When complaints occur, however, even if minor, they can be bothersome to the pregnant woman. Peripheral nerve function may threaten the mother and fetus in various ways during gestation. Quick recognition and treatment efforts should therefore be the clinician's goal.

Mononeuropathies

Many mononeuropathies occur during pregnancy. The following discussion divides them by location.

Cranial nerves

Facial nerve

Bell palsy, the most common disorder of the facial nerve and of idiopathic etiology [1], has a slightly higher incidence of involvement in women. The risk for developing Bell palsy during pregnancy or directly after gestation is three times higher than in nonpregnant women. The third trimester or the 2 weeks immediately postpartum is most common [2].

Hypertension, gestational edema, viral infections, and hypercoagulability are suggested etiologies. Hypertensive disorders during pregnancy are more frequent, because they occur in Bell palsy [3].

The course of Bell palsy during pregnancy is similar to that seen in all cases. There is sudden weakness of the entire ipsilateral face and sometimes subjective numbness. No objective sensory loss is found. The patients rarely

* Corresponding author.
  E-mail address: stolp.kathryn@mayo.edu (K.A. Stolp).

have bilateral involvement; however, they may have ear pain, hyperacusis, and absence of taste ipsilaterally. Onset of maximum weakness is within hours to days. When some motor function is preserved it is a good prognostic sign. Complete or near complete recovery of facial strength occurs in most cases. Recurrence of Bell palsy in subsequent pregnancies is unusual.

Electrophysiologic studies can be useful during this period. They may be helpful in predicting recovery. Facial stimulation as a therapeutic measure has not been consistently demonstrated to be helpful in recovery.

Treatment of Bell palsy includes prednisone for a short course and acyclovir [4]. Obviously this is of less risk when it occurs in the third trimester or postpartum period insofar as causing harm to the fetus. When patients are treated with steroids, blood pressure and blood glucose levels must be monitored closely. The eye must be lubricated to protect the cornea from abrasions, and recovery during pregnancy seems to be at the same rate as in nonpregnant patients. Residual problems from this paralysis include incomplete recovery, facial synkinesis, and crocodile tears.

Auditory nerves

On rare occasions, women during pregnancy lose their ability to hear. This seems to be vascular in etiology and can be severe. The exact etiology has not been determined and prognostication is difficult. Women often require head MRI evaluation to rule out a cerebellopontine angle tumor or other compressive etiology. Viral etiologies also occur.

Oculomotor nerve

Diplopia may occur in pregnant women, but it is rare. It may occur with cranial nerve III involvement and may be transient. Persistent isolated paresis should prompt a search for causes, as it would in any nonpregnant woman. Obviously, cranial nerve III involvement with pupil sparing would suggest nerve infarctions, such as occurs in diabetes mellitus, and pupillotonia might suggest aneurysm involving the posterior communicating artery. This is not unique to pregnancy, however.

Myasthenia gravis may present during pregnancy with external ocular muscle dysfunction and may mimic isolated muscle paresis. Involvement of the cranial nerve IV is extremely uncommon in pregnancy and is rarely caused by a structural abnormality.

Abducens nerve

Diplopia may occur during pregnancy because of an abducens nerve (VI) palsy from elevated intracranial pressure, such as that seen in idiopathic intracranial hypertension. Abrupt hypertension can cause increased intracranial pressure and VI nerve palsy. This may also be seen in pre-eclampsia. It may occur postpartum, and if associated with headaches or focal symptoms, one might be concerned with sinus thrombosis [5].

Optic nerve

Visual loss during pregnancy is rare. Optic neuritis (retrobulbar; disc edema) may occur during pregnancy, particularly in the second trimester, and may produce visual loss and subsequent optic atrophy. This can be bilateral and severe. The clinician should be concerned for possibility of demyelinating disease. Idiopathic intracranial hypertension causing visual loss, although uncommon in pregnancy, is important to recognize and manage, even with shunt procedures.

Neuroimaging is important in this situation to evaluate for orbital apex masses, such as meningioma, glioma, or aneurysmal compression, and to look for more diffuse evidence of demyelinating plaques. Aneurysms and meningiomas sometimes enlarge during pregnancy.

Upper extremities

Median nerve and carpal tunnel syndrome

Carpal tunnel syndrome is a frequent problem in pregnancy. Key presenting features are pain at night with sensory disturbance in a median nerve distribution. Clinical findings may include loss of sensation and thenar atrophy or weakness in a median nerve distribution. One of the challenges is distinguishing carpal tunnel syndrome from hand discomfort in pregnancy. It is estimated that 30% to 35% of all pregnant women have hand discomfort during pregnancy at one point in the gestation. What distinguishes this from carpal tunnel syndrome is that it is most often bilateral, it is not in a specific nerve distribution, and usually there is less burning and no night pain [6–10].

The etiology of carpal tunnel syndrome in pregnancy is not completely understood. It is known that the incidence is higher in nonpregnant females than in males. Whether this is attributable to a smaller carpal canal, hormonal differences that occur during pregnancy, or degree of adipose tissue is not clear. The incidence is also higher in perimenopausal women. This is believed to relate to increased fluid retention, the effects of relaxin and other hormonal changes on ligamentous laxity, altered amounts of adipose tissue, and perhaps to altered sleep position [11–16]. Butterworth and colleagues [17] found increased sensitivity to a lidocaine block in pregnant women, and this may imply changes in the nerve itself during pregnancy. Another important point is the incidence of carpal tunnel syndrome that occurs in the postpartum period. This is most typically associated with individuals who are breastfeeding and is believed to be caused by awkward positions often necessary to successfully breastfeed [18].

Stevens and colleagues [19] found that up to 50% of pregnant women have some nocturnal symptoms in the third trimester. Of those who have carpal tunnel syndrome, 2.3% to 4.6% are pregnant, and in the 15- to 44-year age group, carpal tunnel syndrome is two to three times more frequent in pregnant than nonpregnant females. Stolp-Smith and colleagues [20] found in a large retrospective study of 10,873 women who experienced

14,579 pregnancies in Olmsted County, Minnesota, that in less than 1% who had carpal tunnel syndrome recorded in the medical record, 8% of the cases occurred in the first trimester, 32% in the second trimester, and 35% in the third trimester. There was no correlation with weight gain, onset and gestation interval, or pre-eclampsia. Symptoms in these patients were typically paresthesias, which were bilateral in 68%, and pain in 67%, with a positive median Tinel sign in 95%. Most had some degree of generalized edema by the third trimester.

Melvin and colleagues [21] performed serial nerve conduction studies in pregnant women. No changes were seen in the control group of asymptomatic women. In pregnant women, 7% had prolonged median motor or sensory distal latencies. Findings returned to normal as early as the eighth month of pregnancy or as late as 10 months postpartum. Seror [6] studied 52 carpal tunnel syndrome hands in 30 pregnancies. More than 20 demonstrated motor or sensory "conduction blocks" and 5 had "severe denervation changes." Prospective median and ulnar nerve conduction studies matched by age and parity to control subjects found prolonged medial distal latencies in the pregnant group, more so in those with symptoms, and that the inter-palmar latency was the best comparison for positive electrodiagnosis [22].

Given the high likelihood that carpal tunnel symptoms resolve in the immediate postpartum period, management is typically conservative. Avoiding aggravating factors, which includes taking a thorough history of occupational and other activities of daily living, wearing wrist hand orthoses, and controlling edema, are all important. Beyond that, it is not clear if it is necessary to use modalities or injections or to pursue surgery. Attention should be given to postpartum activities if there are persistent symptoms, and in particular if surgery is performed; this may have implications for positional changes in hand and arm use in the postpartum period. Al Qattan reported that 76% of carpal tunnel resolved 1 month postpartum. Ninety-three percent of pregnant patients ceased nocturnal awakening from pain, and seven women required surgery 2 to 16 years later [8]. Wand [18] noted that 40% of pregnant women who had carpal tunnel syndrome who were followed had signs but not symptoms of median nerve dysfunction postpartum. It is believed that conservative therapy may fail if symptom onset is before pregnancy or if it occurs in the first two trimesters. Also, a positive Phalen sign within 30 seconds and abnormal two-point discrimination combined indicate a poor prognosis for response to conservative treatment.

In summary, carpal tunnel syndrome in pregnancy has a higher incidence than in the general population, and the etiology is uncertain. Symptoms are more severe than the typical hand pain in pregnancy. Electrodiagnosis can be used to differentiate between pregnancy hand pain and carpal tunnel syndrome. Conservative treatment is usually successful. Care should be taken in the postpartum period to avoid activities and postures that could aggravate carpal tunnel syndrome, and patients should be reassured that most have resolution of symptoms in the immediate postpartum period.

Ulnar nerve

Sensory distribution in the medial (ulnar) aspect of the palm dorsally and ventrally with sensory dysfunction and pain occur infrequently during pregnancy and certainly less commonly than median involvement. The ulnar nerve is most commonly injured at the olecranon groove or in the cubital tunnel. Sometimes it may be involved more distally at Guyon canal. Search for some traumatic mechanism is of value in this situation, as is the association of women having previous fractures of their proximal radius ("tardy ulnar palsy").

Electrophysiologic diagnosis may be extremely helpful in localizing the etiology of the involvement to the wrist, elbow, or even in between. Involvement bilaterally must be ruled out, and the clinician must be sure that there is not more diffuse involvement of the nerves with only symptoms localized to the ulnar distribution.

Therapy usually involves care to not traumatize the olecranon groove or other site of compression [23].

Brachial plexus

Idiopathic brachial plexus involvement and hereditary brachial plexus neuropathy may occur in the postpartum period and less frequently during pregnancy. Some re-occur in subsequent pregnancies. Early, there is pain in the shoulder and upper arm, followed by weakness, atrophy, and occasional localized isolated axillary sensory loss.

Most of these patients recover, but this may take up to 2 to 3 years [24].

Electrodiagnostic tests may be performed to confirm the diagnosis. Usually axonal damage is a predominant feature.

Lower extremities

Peroneal nerve

This peroneal neuropathy during pregnancy is rare, except in the situation of trauma at delivery. Weakness in the anterior compartment muscles or paresthesias in the anterolateral part of the leg would prompt the clinician to evaluate for this etiology, particularly if no low back pain or radicular symptoms are present. Most common concern is trauma at the fibular head and neck, but neuromas and cysts may also localize to this area [23]. Electrodiagnostic tests and ultrasound may help determine the etiology or localize the level of the lesion.

Tibial nerve

Tibial nerve may be involved with various reports of tarsal tunnel syndrome during pregnancy. There is pain at the ankle and foot and paresthesias over the sole of the foot, just inferior to the medial malleolus. With increasing edema during pregnancy, local trauma is a concern similar to problems that occur in nonpregnant women. The symptoms often abate after delivery [25,26].

Involvement at the tibial nerve in the popliteal fossa must be distinguished from tarsal tunnel syndrome; this is best done by electrodiagnostic studies. Baker cyst in the popliteal fossa has been known to produce symptoms during pregnancy from enlargement.

Lumbosacral plexus

Involvement of the lumbosacral plexus may rarely develop during the third trimester and is suspected to be caused by compression from the fetus. Rarely, a lumbosacral plexopathy occurs during pregnancy as part of hereditary brachial plexus neuropathy. Usually involvement of the plexus resolves well following delivery [27].

Electrodiagnostic tests are invaluable to help determine the extent of the involvement, prognostic issues, and to rule out other etiologies, such as radicular involvement.

Lateral femoral cutaneous nerve of the thigh

Numbness and paresthesias in the anterolateral thigh and sometimes significant pain may result from damage to the lateral femoral cutaneous nerve. Known as "meralgia paresthetica," this occurs during pregnancy, most commonly in the third trimester. Location of the involvement of the nerve has been associated with at least nine specific possible points of compression along the route. Most likely increased abdominal size and weight gain may cause stretch injury to the nerve and may alter the angle of the nerve at various locations, including the inguinal ligament or as the nerve enters or exits the tensor fossa lata.

Electrodiagnostic tests are rarely needed during this situation, but they can be performed. Usually this is a clinical diagnosis, often with resolution of symptoms postpartum [23].

Medical treatment during pregnancy, beyond reassurance, may include lidocaine patches. With severe pain, oral medications can be considered after the third trimester. Anesthetic injections sometimes are used.

Intercostal and abdominal nerves

Intercostal neuralgia can occur in the last trimester of pregnancy and is usually believed to be caused by a stretch injury of the intercostal nerves from a large fetus or some mechanical cause. There is usually mild pain, but it is sometimes severe and follows the distribution of one or two thoracic roots. Epidural anesthesia may rarely be needed for disabling cases; this usually resolves following delivery and seldom recurs. Obviously if skin shows a rash, one must consider herpes zoster. Thoracoradiculopathy in patients who have diabetes mellitus may cause similar pain [28].

Electrodiagnostic tests are rarely required, because this is a clinical diagnosis. Localized paraspinal neurogenic changes may be found in some but are rarely required to make the diagnosis.

Sensory mononeuropathy

Several parestheticas occur in women that may present during pregnancy [23]. Meralgia paresthetica (lateral femoral cutaneous nerve of the thigh) has been discussed. It may arise during pregnancy. Sometimes pre-existing involvement may worsen symptoms. Cheralgia paresthetica (superficial radial nerve), gonyalgia paresthetica (prepatellar branch of saphenous nerve), digitalgia paresthetica (digital nerve), and nostalgia paresthetica (dorsal primary roots of T2–6) may become symptomatic while a women is pregnant. Generally these are pre-existing and resolve after delivery. Usually reassurance to the mother is all that is needed.

Polyneuropathy

Autoimmune neuropathies

Acute immune demyelinating polyneuropathy

Acute or subacute motor neuropathy with a monophasic course is seen during pregnancy (acute immune demyelinating polyneuropathy [AIDP] or Guillain-Barre syndrome) [29]. Although generally considered an ascending symmetric weakness with paresthesias, strength may be lost proximally greater than distally on some occasions. Reflexes are usually lost, except in early cases, and spinal fluid demonstrates the cytoalbuminologic dissociation. Sensation is usually spared on examination despite the profound weakness.

Electrophysiologic studies are important, but early on they may be fairly normal. Later they typically show prolonged F-wave latencies, then slowed conduction velocities and prolonged distal latencies.

AIDP during pregnancy has a similar incidence to the nonpregnant state. Women may develop this weakness at any time during the pregnancy, but most commonly in the third trimester. This is an immune-mediated illness, but viral syndromes do precede onset in almost two thirds of all cases. Screening for cytomegalic virus, Epstein Barr virus, HIV, *Campylobacter jejune*, varicella zoster, and other viral infections may be performed.

During late gestation, respiratory decompensation may occur because of diminished lung volumes and an elevated diaphragm and may restrict the mother's vital capacity [30]. The respiratory function should be serially evaluated to follow the mother's course. When mechanical ventilation is required, the mother may be at higher risk for premature labor, thromboembolic complications, respiratory distress, or even sepsis.

Treatment is multifaceted and includes good nutrition, prevention of embolic complications, observation for autonomic dysfunction, and good fluid management. Plasmapheresis or intravenous immune globulin is effective in nonpregnant patients and can be used safely during pregnancy [31].

Because AIDP has no effect on uterine contraction, patients may undergo vaginal delivery. These patients, however, are considered an at-risk group of women. Respiratory and pain control and general anesthesia issues should be maintained carefully by the anesthesiologist. The fetal survival rate is 96%.

Chronic immune demyelinating polyneuropathy

A chronic form of demyelinating polyneuropathy (CIDP) involves sensory and motor neuropathy of autoimmune character. The onset may be more subacute, occurring over months, and sometimes it may take on a relapsing course. The incidence of relapse may increase during pregnancy or the patient may worsen and may be progressively weak during the third trimester or postpartum period [32].

Treatment considerations include plasmapheresis, intravenous Ig (IVIg), and possibly even steroids [33]. Women who have known CIDP on immunosuppression who wish to become pregnant should be educated about the risks for herself and the fetus and perhaps switch to less harmful agents prophylactically.

Multifocal motor neuropathy

Some patients who have multifocal motor neuropathy (MMN) may worsen and have increased weakness during pregnancy [34]. The occurrence of this association is infrequent and cases are rare, but some have shown previously unaffected muscles becoming weak during pregnancy. MMN is most likely a humerally related mediated disease with antibodies to gangliosides (GM-I, GM-II, and GDI-A). The patients usually respond to IVIg.

Metabolic polyneuropathies

Diabetes mellitus

Diabetic neuropathy is a diffuse distal chronic sensorimotor neuropathy. There are other manifestations seen in patients who have diabetes mellitus, which include diabetic amyotrophy, autonomic neuropathy, and thoracolumbar radiculopathy. These may be more frequent in diabetic women during pregnancy [35]. Neuropathy caused by diabetes mellitus does not necessarily worsen during pregnancy and is seldom a major issue of concern, other than the mother's discomfort [36,37].

Postpartum the incidence of peripheral neuropathy may increase, perhaps as much as tenfold [37]. This suggests that the neuropathy during pregnancy can worsen in certain situations, particularly with insulin-dependent diabetes. Electrophysiologic tests have failed to demonstrate induction or worsening; however, there does seem to be a direct correlation with glycemic control.

Electrophysiologic abnormalities show slowed nerve conductions with reduced amplitudes. Sometimes when small-fiber neuropathy is predominant, they are normal.

Porphyria

Hepatic porphyria occurs in young women and occasionally occurs while they are pregnant [38]. Acute intermittent porphyria, variac porphyria, or even hereditary porphyria have enzymatic defects that affect the keen synthesis pathway. Precipitating factors then may lead to excessive production of porphobilinogen or delta aminolevulinic acid in young women. Oral contraceptives during the menstrual cycle may produce exacerbations of neuropathy or other symptoms, including psychiatric disturbance or abdominal pain. In a young woman known to have porphyria, proper medication during the pregnancy is essential to prevent an attack. Elimination of exacerbating medications and giving glucose and carbohydrate meals should be instituted as treatment. Sometimes treatment with hematin prevents subsequent neurologic problems [23].

Electrodiagnostic testing assists in determining the severity and prognosis and usually shows a diffuse sensorimotor and sometimes autonomic neuropathy.

Nutritional neuropathies

Gestational women on occasion have marginal nutritional status or hyperemesis gravidarum that can develop into vitamin deficiency. This may involve thiamine, vitamin B6, or sometimes other vitamins. Specifically a sensorimotor neuropathy occasionally develops from thiamine deficiency and may occur even without encephalopathy. This is usually an asymmetric axonal neuropathy and may be demonstrated by electrophysiologic studies [23].

Treatment is intravenous thiamine and as soon as the patient is able, promotion of a better diet with oral thiamine. This neuropathy usually improves quickly with proper treatment.

Toxic neuropathies

Toxins may cause neuropathy in various situations. Those associated with pregnancy often are related to iatrogenic or medical therapy.

Nitrofurantoin, even without renal involvement, may cause an axonal sensorimotor neuropathy when it is used for treatment of urinary tract infections during pregnancy. Symptoms may be profound and may not immediately dissipate following discontinuing the medications. There is also the concern that the fetus may develop some neuropathies in association with nitrofurantoin therapy if given early in the first trimester [23].

Since recognition of fetal thalidomide toxicity in the 1950s, restricted use of any drug, including nitrofurantoin, is suggested to reduce the exposure of the fetus.

Hereditary polyneuropathy

Charcot-Marie-Tooth (CMT) is a demyelinating neuropathy that may have exacerbations during pregnancy. Women who develop symptoms earlier in life are more prone to exacerbations during pregnancy, and temporary worsening occurs in approximately one third of patients [39]. Steroids are not proven efficacious in CMT I but have been reported to help symptoms in one case. The obvious issues of difficulty with ambulation must be watched during this period to prevent falls and other risky situations. Cases of CMT II in pregnancy have been rare.

Electrodiagnostic tests, if not performed earlier, may confirm this diagnosis. Genetic testing or ultrasound on some nerves may be beneficial when needed to confirm diagnosis.

Labor and delivery

During labor and delivery, acute neuropathies may occur that involve the lumbosacral plexus, spinal nerve roots, or even the peripheral nerves. Because of awareness of common compression sites, the incidence of this form of neuropathy has declined.

Lumbosacral plexopathy

This plexopathy occurs during active labor or in the third trimester and produces pelvic or proximal leg weakness and pain, most often affecting L4 and L5 innervated muscles, producing weakness of dorsiflexion and foot eversion and inversion. Often the Achilles reflex is preserved and sensory impairment predominates in the L5 dermatome.

Electrodiagnostic tests show a demyelinating lesion in the lumbosacral trunk area, sparing the paraspinal muscles [40].

The occurrence of the lumbosacral plexopathy may be caused by the fetal head at the pelvic brim where the nerve is unprotected. The differential diagnosis includes lumbar disc herniation, spinal root damage from an epidural anesthesia, and occasionally local trauma from care given during the labor. Risk factors for its occurrence include protracted labor, cephalopelvic disproportion, large gestational weight, and maternal short stature. Most patients recover in the months following delivery.

Femoral neuropathy

Femoral neuropathy may become symptomatic during labor or immediately postpartum. It complicates the postpartum period because of unilateral or bilateral involvement most often, but it can occur during the third trimester [41].

Patients have trouble standing, difficulty climbing stairs, and sometimes sensory loss in the anteromedial thigh. Examination reveals reduced knee reflex and weakness of the quadriceps femoris and the iliopsoas with sensory loss in the medial part of the thigh. If the iliopsoas is weak, injury is proximal to the inguinal ligament, but when limited to the quadriceps femoris, it may be at the inguinal ligament. Fetal compression and stretch injury by excessive hip abduction and external rotation or even occasionally instrumentation during delivery may cause injury. The differential diagnosis includes retroperitoneal hemorrhage or intrapelvic pathology.

Electrodiagnostic tests are often not required if resolution occurs quickly, but if symptoms persist, these can be invaluable to rule out other etiologies than that limited to the femoral nerve. MRI of the pelvis or ultrasound is often warranted.

Obturator neuropathy

Protracted labor may also cause an obturator neuropathy by nerve compression between the fetal head and bony pelvic wall, exacerbated by external rotation and abduction of the thighs. Women report leg weakness while walking, pain in the groin and upper thigh, or paresthesias along the medial thigh.

Symptoms may be transient. The diagnosis is often unrecognized. Weakness of thigh adduction, sensory deficit over the proximal medial thigh, and a circumducting gait are found. Normal knee reflex and quadriceps femoris strength help eliminate plexus lesions or L3 or L4 radiculopathies.

Vaginal examination and imaging studies can exclude compression from hematoma or tumor. Women generally recover completely, and residual neuropathic pain does occur [42].

Peroneal neuropathy

Following labor, women may report paresthesias along the anterior lateral aspect of the leg and may notice difficulty with dorsiflexion of the foot. Examination shows problems with dorsiflexion, toe extension, and eversion, and may sometimes be limited to the superficial branch of the peroneal nerve, just the deep branch of the peroneal nerve, or both branches, because the common peroneal cross the fibular head and neck. At this location, pressure on the peroneal nerve by manual compression can sometimes cause an uncomfortable situation [43]. It may be caused by the stirrups or other mechanical injury during prolonged pressure in this location. Prognosis is good for recovery, but patients must avoid repetitive pressure in this location. Assistance devices may be required for a period of time to assist in ambulation.

Electrophysiologic testing may be important to distinguish this location from lumbosacral plexopathy or an L5 radiculopathy, unless the clinical symptoms and signs are so typical that that may be a deciding factor. Ultrasound may help.

Ilioinguinal, genital femoral, and iliohypogastric neuropathy

Stretch injury or nerve entrapment following Pfannenstiel incision may produce lower abdominal, inguinal, or upper thigh pain and sometimes dysesthesias. These are sensory abnormalities produced by involvement of the ilioinguinal and genital femoral nerve on the skin overlying the lower abdomen, upper medial thigh, inguinal ligament, labor majora, and mons pubis. In addition, iliohypogastric involvement may cause sensory dysfunction above the pubis and upper buttocks and sometimes involving the lower abdominal muscles. These symptoms are sensory only and involve no motor involvement. The symptoms usually resolve if they are caused by a stretch injury.

Electrodiagnostic tests are not usually helpful, because this is a clinical diagnosis. Therapeutic nerve blocks may decrease the pain and Lidoderm patches may be helpful.

Pudendal neuropathy

Large episiotomies and local tissue damage from prolonged fetal compression may injure the pudendal nerve, producing numbness and incontinence [44]. Following delivery, women may develop urinary stress incontinence or fecal incontinence later in life. Sphincter injury, pelvic floor descent, and accumulative nerve damage from stretch injury following labor all may be involved in producing symptoms.

Electrophysiologic studies include anal sphincter EMG demonstrating neuropathic changes in the anal sphincter, and sometimes pudendal nerve latencies may be helpful. Ultrasound evaluation is of unknown advantage at this time.

Therapy involves surgical repair of the anal sphincter, which has variable ability to produce continence [45].

References

[1] Katusic SK, Beard CM, Wiederholt WC, et al. Incidence, clinical features, and prognosis in Bell's palsy, Rochester, Minnesota, 1968–1982. Ann Neurol 1986;20:622–7.

[2] Falco NA, Eriksson E. Idiopathic facial palsy in pregnancy and the puerperium. Surg Gynecol Obstet 1989;169(4):337–40.

[3] Shmorgun D, Chan WS, Ray JG. Association of Bell's palsy in pregnancy and preeclampsia. QJM 2002;95:359–62.

[4] Grogan PM, Gronseth PM. Practice parameter: steroids, acyclovir, and surgery for Bell's palsy (an evidence based medicine review): report on the Quality Standards Subcommittee of the American Academy of Neurology. Neurology 2001;56:830–6.

[5] Barry-Kinsella C, Milner M, McCarthy N, et al. Sixth nerve palsy: an unusual manifestation of preeclampsia. Obstet Gynecol 1994;83:849–51.

[6] Seror P. Pregnancy-related carpal tunnel syndrome. J Hand Surg [Br] 1998;23:98–101.

[7] Dekel S, Papaioannou T, Rushworth G, et al. Idiopathic carpal tunnel syndrome caused by carpal stenosis. BMJ 1980;280:1297–9.

[8] al Qattan MM, Manktelow RT, Bowen CV. Pregnancy-induced carpal tunnel syndrome requiring surgical release longer than 2 years after delivery. Obstet Gynecol 1994;84:249–51.

[9] Graham RA. Carpal tunnel syndrome: a statistical analysis of 214 cases. Orthopedics 1983;6: 1283–7.

[10] Weiss AP, Akelman E. Carpal tunnel syndrome: a review. R I Med 1992;75:303–6.

[11] Ekman-Ordeberg G, Salgeback S, Ordeberg G. Carpal tunnel syndrome in pregnancy. A prospective study. Acta Obstet Gynecol Scand 1987;66:233–5.

[12] McLennan HG, Oats JN, Walstab JE. Survey of hand symptoms in pregnancy. Med J Aust 1987;147:542–4.

[13] Vessey MP, Villard-Mackintosh L, Yeates D. Epidemiology of carpal tunnel syndrome in women of childbearing age. Findings in a large cohort study. Int J Epidemiol 1990;19:655–9.

[14] Hagberg M, Morgenstern H, Kelsh M. Impact of occupations and job tasks on the prevalence of carpal tunnel syndrome. Scan J Work Environ Health 1992;18:337–45.

[15] Radecki P. Personal factors and blood volume movement in causation of median neuropathy at the carpal tunnel. Am J Phys Med Rehabil 1996;75:235–8.

[16] Werner RA, Albers JW, Franzblau A, et al. The relationship between body mass index and the diagnosis of carpal tunnel syndrome. Muscle Nerve 1994;17:632–6.

[17] Butterworth JF IV, Walker FO, Lysak SZ. Pregnancy increases median nerve susceptibility to lidocaine. Anesthesiology 1990;72:962–5.

[18] Wand JS. Carpal tunnel syndrome in pregnancy and lactation. J Hand Surg [Br] 1990;15: 93–5.

[19] Stevens JC, Beard CM, O'Fallon WM, et al. Conditions associated with carpal tunnel syndrome. Mayo Clin Proc 1992;67:541–8.

[20] Stolp-Smith KA, Pascoe MK, Ogburn PL. Carpal tunnel syndrome in pregnancy: frequency, severity, and prognosis. Arch Phys Med Rehabil 1998;79:1285–7.

[21] Melvin JL, Burnett CN, Johnson EW. Median nerve conduction in pregnancy. Arch Phys Med Rehabil 1969;50:75–80.

[22] Eogan M, O'Brien C, Carolan D, et al. Median and ulnar nerve conduction in pregnancy. Int J Gynaecol Obstet 2004;87(3):233–6.

[23] Moore A, Massey EW, Massey J. Peripheral nerve disease in women. In: Kaplan PW, editor. Neurologic disease in women. 2nd edition. New York: Demos Medical Publishing, Inc; 2006.

[24] Tsairis P, Dyck PJ, Mulder DW. Natural history of brachial plexus neuropathy: report on 99 patients. Arch Neurol 1972;27:109–17.

[25] Massey EW. Mononeuropathies in pregnancy. Semin Neurol 1988;8:193–6.

[26] Rhodes P. Meralgia paresthetica in pregnancy. Lancet 1957;2:831.

[27] Delarue MW, Vles JS, Hassaart TH. Lumbosacral plexopathy in the third trimester of pregnancy: a report of three cases. Eur J Obstet Gynecol Reprod Biol 1994;53:67–8.

[28] Pleet AB, Massey EW. Intercostal neuralgia of pregnancy. JAMA 1980;243:770.

[29] Jiang GX, de Pedro-Cuesta J, Strigard K, et al. Pregnancy and Guillain-Barre syndrome: a nationwide register cohort study. Neuroepidemiology 1996;15:192–200.

[30] Ropper AR, Wijdicks EFM, Traux BT. Guillain-barre syndrome. Philadelphia: FA Davis; 1991.

[31] Nelson LH, Maclean WT. Management of Landry-Guillain-Barre syndrome in pregnancy. Obstet Gynecol 1985;65:S25–9.

[32] Barohn RJ, Kissel JT, Warmolts JR, et al. Chronic inflammatory demyelinating polyradiculoneuropathy. Clinical characteristics, course, and recommendations for diagnostic criteria. Arch Neurol 1989;46:878–84.

[33] Dyck PJ, Daube J, O'Brien P, et al. Plasma exchange in chronic inflammatory demyelinating polyneuropathy. N Engl J Med 1986;314:461–5.

[34] Chaudry V, Escolar DM, Cornblath DR. Worsening of multifocal motor neuropathy during pregnancy. Neurology 2002;59:139–41.

[35] Hemachandra A, Ellis D, Lloyd CE, et al. The influence of pregnancy on IDDM complications. Diabetes Care 1995;18:950–4.

[36] Lapolla A, Cardone C, Negrin P, et al. Pregnancy does not induce or worsen retinal or peripheral nerve dysfunction in insulin-dependent diabetic women. J Diabetes Complicat 1998;12:74–80.

[37] Diabetes Control and Complications Trial Research Group. The effect of intensive diabetes therapy on the development and progression of neuropathy. Ann Intern Med 1995;122: 561–8.

[38] Vine S, Shaffer HM, Pauley G, et al. A review of the relationship between pregnancy and porphyria and presentation of a case. Ann Intern Med 1957;47:834–40.

[39] Rudnik-Schoneborn S, Rohrig D, Nicholson G, et al. Pregnancy and delivery in Charcot-Marie-Tooth disease type 1. Neurology 1993;43:2011–6.

[40] Katirji B, Wilbourn AJ, Scarberry SL, et al. Intrapartum maternal lumbosacral plexopathy. Muscle Nerve 2002;26:340–7.

[41] Dar AQ, Robinson A, Lyons G. Postpartum femoral neuropathy: more common than you think. Anesthesia 1999;54:512.

[42] Warfield CA. Obturator neuropathy after forceps delivery. Obstet Gynecol 1984;64:47S–8S.

[43] Adornato BT, Carlini WG. "Pushing palsy:" a case of self-induced bilateral peroneal palsy during natural childbirth. Neurology 1992;42:936–7.

[44] Fitzpatrick M, O'Herlihy C. The effects of labour and delivery on the pelvic floor. Best Pract Res Clin Obstet Gynaecol 2001;15:63–79.

[45] Sangwan YP, Coller JA, Barrett RC, et al. Unilateral pudendal neuropathy. Impact on outcome of anal sphincter repair. Dis Colon Rectum 1996;39:686–9.

ELSEVIER
SAUNDERS

Phys Med Rehabil Clin N Am
19 (2008) 163–194

PHYSICAL MEDICINE
AND REHABILITATION
CLINICS OF
NORTH AMERICA

Musculoskeletal Complications of Neuromuscular Disease in Children

Sherilyn W. Driscoll, MD[a,b,*], Joline Skinner, MD[a]

[a]Pediatric Physical Medicine and Rehabilitation, Mayo Clinic,
200 First Street SW, Rochester, MN 55901, USA
[b]Mayo Clinic College of Medicine, 200 First Street SW, Rochester, MN, 55901 USA

A wide variety of neuromuscular diseases affect children, including central nervous system disorders such as cerebral palsy and spinal cord injury; motor neuron disorders such as spinal muscular atrophy; peripheral nerve disorders such as Charcot-Marie-Tooth disease; neuromuscular junction disorders such as congenital myasthenia gravis; and muscle fiber disorders such as Duchenne's muscular dystrophy. Although the origins and clinical syndromes vary significantly, outcomes related to musculoskeletal complications are often shared. The most frequently encountered musculoskeletal complications of neuromuscular disorders in children are scoliosis, bony rotational deformities, and hip dysplasia. Management is often challenging to those who work with children who have neuromuscular disorders.

Scoliosis

Scoliosis refers to deviation from normal spinal alignment. A commonly accepted definition of scoliosis is a curvature in the coronal plane of greater than 10°. The coronal curvature is almost always associated with a sagittal alignment abnormality, such as kyphosis, lordosis, or a rotational component. Scoliosis may be classified as idiopathic, congenital, or neuromuscular in origin. Overall, idiopathic scoliosis accounts for the significant majority of cases of scoliosis in children and adolescents, whereas scoliosis associated with neuromuscular disease, congenital deformity, and other causes occurs less frequently in the total population. Neuromuscular scoliosis can occur as

* Corresponding author. Pediatric Physical Medicine and Rehabilitation, Mayo Clinic, 200 First Street SW, Rochester, MN 55901.
 E-mail address: driscoll.sherilyn@mayo.edu (S.W. Driscoll).

1047-9651/08/$ - see front matter © 2008 Elsevier Inc. All rights reserved.
doi:10.1016/j.pmr.2007.10.003

a complication of a wide variety of disease processes in children, including upper and lower motor neuron conditions and myopathies.

Scoliosis may lead to functional deficits, such as decreased sitting balance. The upper extremities may be required to maintain upright posture, thereby reducing the availability of the arms for functional daily tasks. Neck, shoulder, and spine range of motion may be limited. In Duchenne's muscular dystrophy, for example, the rigid neck, hyperextension deformity with associated marked increase of cervical lordosis forces patients to bend their trunk forward and assume an awkward posture to look straight ahead [1]. Scoliosis may result in skin breakdown or pain. As scoliosis becomes more severe, reduction in lung volumes and diaphragmatic heights may occur [2]. Beyond 100°, pulmonary hypertension and right ventricular hypertrophy may develop [3].

Epidemiology

Idiopathic scoliosis occurs in 2% to 3% of the adolescent population [4]. In contrast, the rates of spinal deformity in children who have neuromuscular disease are generally much higher and depend on the diagnosis (Table 1). For example, 20% of patients who have mild cerebral palsy may develop scoliosis, but nearly 100% of those who have thoracic spinal cord injury that occurs before puberty will develop this disease. Although idiopathic scoliosis is much more common in girls than boys [26], neuromuscular scoliosis does not discriminate between the genders. Children who have undergone selective dorsal rhizotomy for spasticity control seem to have a higher incidence of spinal deformity than those who have not undergone this procedure [27–30].

Origin

The origin of idiopathic scoliosis is unknown, although genetic, environmental, and undetected neuromuscular dysfunction are hypothesized causes [29,30]. In neuromuscular scoliosis, the situation is even more complex.

Table 1
Prevalence of scoliosis and hip dysplasia in children who have neuromuscular disease

	Cerebral palsy	Myelomeningocele	Duchenne's muscular dystrophy	Spinal cord injury	Charcot-Marie-Tooth	Spinal muscular atrophy
Scoliosis	38%–64% [5,6]	20%–94% [7]	63%–90% [8,9]	100% [10] (if injured before adolescent growth spurt)	10% [11]	70%–100% [12–14]
Hip dysplasia	2%–60% [15–18]	1%–28% [19]	35% [20]	29%–82% [21–23]	6%–8% [24]	11%–38% [25]

Upright posture may be impaired because of abnormalities in the intricate coordination among central nervous system, muscle, bone, cartilage, and soft tissue. Asymmetric weakness, spasticity, abnormal sensory feedback, or mechanical factors such as pelvic obliquity or unilateral hip dislocation may cause an initial, flexible spinal curve. However, which parameter contributes most or even determines the direction of the curve is still unknown. No significant correlation between muscle asymmetry or side of dislocated hip and side of scoliotic convexity has been discovered [7,15]. Whatever the origin or initial trigger, once a postural abnormality is present, a vicious cycle of progression may occur such that unequal compression on vertebrae causes unequal growth. Asymmetric growth may cause further unequal compression on the spinal structures, causing the cycle to perpetuate itself. If this cycle is sustained beyond a critical threshold of weight and time, fixed deformity with changes in vertebral and rib structure may follow, and spinal deformity develops [31]. Various triggers may cause the imbalanced spinal axis, but biomechanical forces may account for its progression [32]. Neuromuscular scoliosis is more likely to be rapidly progressive than idiopathic [11,33]. Some evidence indicates, however, that if the underlying origin is corrected, such as spinal cord untethering, the spinal curvature may improve [34,35].

Evaluation

Many neuromuscular diagnoses are confirmed at or around birth. In those circumstances, subsequent evaluations occur with full knowledge of expected outcomes related to spinal deformity. However, conditions such as the hereditary motor sensory neuropathies may not be recognized until later in childhood, and scoliosis may be the presenting symptom. The history of a child who has scoliosis should include information about pre- and perinatal events; developmental milestones; evidence of skill regression; age of onset of symptoms; other system disorders or anomalies (especially renal and cardiac); the presence of associated symptoms such as sensory loss, weakness, or pain; functional deficits; and family history.

Therefore, idiopathic scoliosis is a diagnosis of exclusion. All children and adolescents who have scoliosis should undergo a careful neurologic and musculoskeletal examination. In one study, 23% of children referred to an orthopedic practice who had scoliosis and an atypical curve, congenital scoliosis, gait abnormality, limb pain, or weakness or foot deformity, had an MRI-identified spinal cord pathology [36]. In children who have no known neuromuscular disease, MRI should be obtained when a rapidly progressive curve (more than 1° per month), left-sided thoracic curve, neurologic deficit, limb deformity, or worrisome pain symptoms are identified.

The physical examination should include evaluation for pelvic obliquity, shoulder girdle asymmetry, waist crease asymmetry, rib prominence, or asymmetry with spinal flexion, leg length discrepancy, fixed foot deformity, hip dislocation or subluxation, and limitation of spinal or extremity range of motion. A full neurologic examination should be performed, including an assessment of strength, muscle tone, reflexes (including abdominal reflexes), sensation, balance, cranial nerve function, speech and language, and cognition. A functional assessment is also an important component. Abnormalities in any of these areas may provide clues to origin, expected outcomes, and treatment strategies.

Radiographic evaluation includes a posteroanterior view of the entire spine. Standing films are most useful, although sitting films may be substituted when necessary. The Cobb method is the most commonly used technique to measure the degree of scoliosis (Fig. 1). A widely accepted grading classification denotes a *mild* curve if between 10° and 40°, a *moderate* curve if between 40° and 65°, and a *severe* curve if greater than 65°. Intra- and interobserver measurement variability is within the range of 3° to 10° for noncongenital scoliosis [37]. Curves are named for the location of the apex vertebrae, and are described as *right* or *left* based on their predominant convexity. They are designated *C-shaped* or *double* depending on their configuration. Idiopathic adolescent curves are more likely to be right-sided and thoracic in location. Experts have believed that neuromuscular curves have a higher incidence of left-sided convexity [11], although a recent retrospective study suggests that the curve patterns and apical levels in neuromuscular scoliosis are similar to those reported for idiopathic adolescent scoliosis

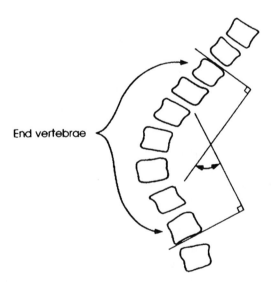

Fig. 1. Cobb method of measuring scoliotic curve in which the vertebra with maximally tilted end plates above and below the apex are identified. The angle between lines drawn along the superior and inferior endplates or the angle of lines drawn perpendicular to them is the Cobb angle. (*From* Magee DJ. Orthopedic physical assessment, 4th edition. Philadelphia: Saunders; 2002. p. 461; with permission.)

[38]. Before surgery, curve flexibility may be assessed using supine lateral bending, fulcrum, or traction radiographs [39].

Nonoperative treatment

If the vicious cycle can be disrupted or the continuous state of asymmetric loading can be prevented early enough that significant spinal bony deformity has not occurred, some experts are hopeful that the progression of scoliosis may be mitigated [40]. A small body of literature suggests that exercise-based approaches in addition to bracing may be effective in some girls who have adolescent idiopathic scoliosis [41–43]. However, the daily use of a spinal orthosis is the mainstay of treatment for girls who have idiopathic scoliosis.

The effectiveness of nonoperative treatment in children who have neuromuscular scoliosis is controversial. Although intuitively attractive, the theory that controlling the mechanical forces acting on the spine will result in decreased curve progression has infrequently been translated into clinical practice [31]. Data are limited regarding efficacy of nonoperative treatment and bracing in preventing curve progression in neuromuscular scoliosis. Olafsson and colleagues [44] reported on brace use in 90 consecutive children who had various types of neuromuscular scoliosis. They observed a 28% success rate (defined as curve progression of less than 10° per year and good brace compliance) with a higher likelihood of improvement in ambulators with hypotonia and short lumbar curves of less than 40° and in nonambulators with spasticity and short lumbar curves. Those who had longer, hypotonic curves experienced less success. In another group of children who had myelomeningocele and a curve not exceeding 45°, a Boston brace was used successfully to arrest or slow the progression of scoliosis in most [45]. However, Miller and colleagues [46] reported no benefit after 67 months of bracing in 20 children who had spastic quadriplegia related to curve magnitude, shape, or rate of progression. Whether spinal orthoses and other conservative management techniques may be helpful in slowing the progression of scoliosis in certain subpopulations of children who have neuromuscular disease remains to be seen, but the prevailing attitude suggests that they are not.

Nonoperative interventions, including sitting supports and custom seating, spinal orthoses, and functional strengthening programs may be useful to improve sitting balance and functional independence [47–50]. In myelodysplasia, a soft thoracolumbosacral orthosis (TLSO) may be used to improve seating and positioning to free the upper extremities for functional tasks or as a temporizing measure to allow the child to develop increased trunk length before surgery [51].

Some are concerned that placing children who have neuromuscular disorders in a TLSO to improve postural function may cause further respiratory compromise, especially for children who have hypotonia. Bayar and colleagues [52] treated 15 children who had neuromuscular scoliosis who used a polyethylene custom spinal orthosis for 8 to 10 hours and postural training, muscle strengthening, and stretching 5 days per week, with special emphasis on respiratory exercises for 4 weeks. Strength, range of motion, and balance improved although scoliosis did not. The forced vital capacity (FVC) while wearing the brace initially decreased by 18%. However, the negative effect on FVC lessened after the program, suggesting an improvement in coping with the restrictive effect of the brace. Further research showed that the use of a soft Boston brace did not impact negatively on the pulmonary mechanics and gas exchange in one group of children who had severe cerebral palsy and, in fact, decreased the work of breathing in some [53].

Special mention of boys who have Duchenne's muscular dystrophy is warranted. Significant progression of scoliosis is unusual while the child remains ambulant. Rapid progression of scoliosis seems to be related to the loss of walking ability and commonly corresponds with a growth spurt in adolescence [54]. The use of corticosteroids [55,56] and orthotics, such as knee-ankle-foot orthoses [57], have been shown to prolong ambulatory ability. This intervention seems to significantly delay onset and decrease severity of scoliosis so that a much smaller proportion of boys who have Duchenne's require surgical stabilization [56,58]. Even without steroid treatment, not all boys who have Duchenne's muscular dystrophy will need scoliosis surgery. It was recently recognized that up to 25% of nonambulant boys do not develop clinically significant scoliosis and therefore do not require surgical intervention [8]. As with other neuromuscular disorders, the primary indication for bracing is to improve postural control and seating rather than prevent progression of curvature [54].

Surgery

The goals of surgical stabilization for spinal deformity in neuromuscular disease include correcting the curvature, preventing significant progression of the curvature, improving the balanced position of the spine, and, therefore, improving quality of life. Indications for surgical intervention include progressive deformity that compromises ability to sit or stand, cardiac or pulmonary function, skin integrity, and ability to perform nursing cares, and causes pain (Fig. 2). Reported outcomes of surgical intervention for neuromuscular scoliosis include improved Cobb angle, lung function, seating position and balance, and ability to perform activities of daily living, and decreased pain and time used for resting (Fig. 3) [59,60]. Self-esteem has also been shown to improve after surgery [60,61]. In Duchenne's muscular dystrophy, most data do not show a significant effect of scoliosis surgery on respiratory function or survival [62,63].

Various surgical techniques have been described and their merits debated. Surgical considerations include anterior and posterior fusion versus posterior-only fusion, one-stage versus two-stage procedures, various instrumentation techniques, and the extension of instrumentation across the

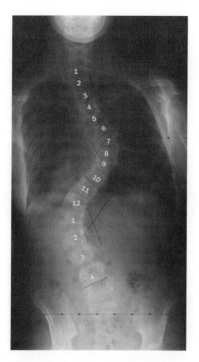

Fig. 2. Preoperative radiograph of an 11-year-old girl who has idiopathic scoliosis.

lumbosacral junction and sacroiliac joint [51,64–66]. From a surgical perspective, best results are achieved when the curve is progressive but not severe or rigid and when medical status is optimal [67].

Children who have neuromuscular scoliosis experience more complicated and costly hospitalizations from their scoliosis surgery than those who have idiopathic scoliosis. Before surgery, children who have neuromuscular disease are more likely to have gastrostomy tubes, failure to thrive, gastroesophageal reflux, and other medical diagnoses. Other challenges related to surgical procedures in children who have neuromuscular disease include curve severity that is characteristically worse and more rigid; osteoporosis; extension of deformity to include fixed pelvic obliquity; poor soft tissue coverage; deficiency of posterior spinal elements, such as in myelodysplasia; and tenuous neurologic status [33,51]. Postoperatively, they experience a higher frequency of pneumonia, respiratory failure, mechanical ventilation, urinary tract infection, surgical wound infection, central line placement, transient or permanent neurologic loss, and failure of the surgical procedure or hardware [51,68,69].

Among children who had cerebral palsy who underwent scoliosis surgery, the number of days in the intensive care unit and the presence of severe preoperative thoracic hyperkyphosis negatively affected survival rate [70]. Negative functional outcomes have been reported, such as loss of ability to roll, feed oneself, and walk [9,61].

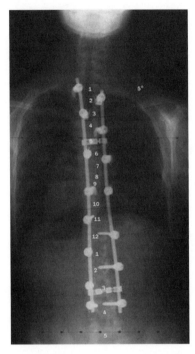

Fig. 3. The same 11-year-old girl as in Fig. 2 who underwent anterior T5–10 fusion with bone graft and posterior T2–L4 fusion with bone graft and Synthes instrumentation.

Historically, children who have severe restrictive lung disease and an FVC of less than 30% of predicted have not been considered surgical candidates. However, several recent studies indicate that with aggressive team management by pulmonary, cardiac, anesthesia, and intensive care pediatric services, these children can safely undergo surgical spine stabilization without the need for tracheostomy or prolonged ventilation [71–73].

Rotational deformities of bone

Rotational malalignment of the lower extremities is a common outcome of neuromuscular disease. The spectrum of bony deformities has been referred to as *lever arm disease* [74,75]. Rotational deformities often occur at the femur and tibia and have a deleterious effect on function and cosmesis. Muscle efficiency may be reduced because the skeletal lever arms are not aligned with the line of progression during gait. For example, in cerebral palsy, intoeing occurs commonly. The increased internal foot progression angle may place muscle groups at a mechanical disadvantage and be associated with poor foot clearance, tripping, and falling and a cosmetically poor gait pattern. Torsional deformities may also be associated with premature degenerative processes at the hip and knee [76–79].

Epidemiology

In a recent retrospective gait analysis study of 412 children who had cerebral palsy, 37% of intoeing gait had multiple causes. The most common contributors, either alone or in combination, were internal hip rotation in 55% and internal tibial torsion in 50%. Pes varus and metatarsus adductus also contributed [80]. Although experts have previously suggested that spasticity of hamstrings and adductors contribute substantially to an internally rotated gait, more recent evidence suggests that intoeing in children who have cerebral palsy is almost universally associated with osseous deformity rather than hypertonia [80–82]. The overall prevalence of excessive internal hip rotation in cerebral palsy is 27%, with prevalence higher in those who have diplegia than in those who have hemiplegia [81].

Etiology

Abnormalities of muscle strength and tone from neuromuscular disease are believed to be ultimately responsible for the development of rotational deformity. Femoral anteversion in able-bodied infants is not significantly different from that in infants who have cerebral palsy. The average newborn shows 30° to 40° of femoral anteversion. This decreases to 10° to 15° by adolescence in a typically developing population [83]. However, children who have cerebral palsy are more likely to experience failure of the typical corrective lateral rotation that occurs with growth and development in their able-bodied counterparts [84]. Persistent hip flexor spasticity and tightness are believed to contribute because they prevent normal extension of the hip and concomitant external rotation, thus the usual remodeling of the infant torsion cannot occur [81].

Similarly, remodeling and lateral derotation of the usual infant internal tibial torsion may not occur in neuromuscular disease. At birth, the malleoli are level in the frontal plane. In typically developing children, most normal external rotation of the tibia occurs by 4 years of age, with an additional degree per year occurring up until skeletal maturity for a final average of 28° of external rotation [85]. Because of this lateral rotation of the tibia that occurs with normal growth, internal rotation abnormalities may improve with time. However, several factors, including muscle imbalance, soft-tissue contractures, associated congenital malformations, and mechanical abnormalities caused by habitually assumed posture over time, may impede this process causing internal tibial torsion to persist. In addition, other children, such as some who have myelomeningocele, may develop significant fixed external tibial torsion associated with valgus of the hindfoot, midfoot abduction, planus deformity, and genu valgum.

Evaluation of lower-extremity rotational deformity

Internal hip rotation, femoral anteversion, and medial femoral torsion all refer to an increased angle of the femoral neck relative to the transcondylar axis of the knee. In other words, the axis of the hip is anterior or external to that of the knee [75]. Femoral anteversion may be assessed using physical examination, radiography, ultrasound, and CT scan and requires optimal positioning of the child for accurate measurement. The most commonly used physical examination maneuver (Craig's test or the Ryder method) places the child prone with pelvis stable, hips extended, and knee flexed to 90°. The leg is then rotated outwardly with goniometric measurement of the angle between the shank and vertical. This angle is equal to the degree of femoral anteversion (Fig. 4).

Tibial torsion is defined as the angle formed between the articular axes of the knee and ankle joint. Tibial torsion is often measured using an assessment of the thigh–foot angle. The child is placed prone with the knee flexed to 90° and the ankle supported in a neutral position. The axis of the foot is then compared with the long axis of the thigh. Alternatively, the degree of tibial torsion can be measured in a seated position, using a goniometer to measure the angle between the visualized bimalleolar axis and the femoral epicondylar axis.

Nonsurgical intervention for torsional deformities

Experts widely believe that traditional exercise, night splints, shoe inserts, twister cables, and other conservative options cannot reverse fixed femoral

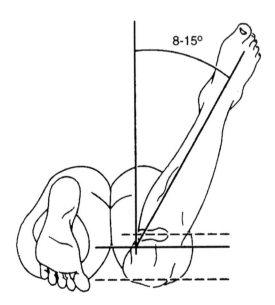

Degree of anteversion

Fig. 4. Prone hip rotation measuring femoral anteversion. (*Adapted from* Magee DJ. Orthopedic physical assessment, 4th edition. Philadelphia: Saunders; 2002. p. 622; with permission.)

or tibial torsion [86]. However, aggressive treatment of spasticity may help prevent development or slow the progression of torsional deformities. Short-term improvements in functional outcomes (gait, Gross Motor Function Measure, and clinical examination) using botulinum toxin injections have been reported, but evidence is limited regarding the effect of botulinum toxin treatment on the development of bony deformity. In a nested case-control design, Desloovere and colleagues [87] reported an improved gait pattern characterized by fewer contractures at the level of the hip, knee, and ankle and decreased internal hip rotation at initial contact, toe-off, and mid-swing in children who had undergone multilevel botulinum A treatments. Botulinum injections were started at a young age and combined with common conservative treatment options. The authors concluded that children treated with multilevel botulinum A injections have a gait pattern less defined by bony deformity than their nontreated counterparts.

Surgery

Medial femoral torsion of greater than 40° to 45° that interferes with gait and function may be corrected surgically with a femoral derotational osteotomy (Figs. 5 and 6). Both proximal and distal surgical techniques have been described. A proximal osteotomy may be beneficial when a child has both femoral torsion and hip subluxation to allow varus angulation of the femoral neck and ensure stability of the hip through proximal femur internal rotation and distal femur external rotation. However, when the hips are stable, distal osteotomies are reportedly less invasive, provide quicker recovery time, and are as effective as proximal surgery in functional and cosmetic outcomes [88–90]. They also provide the added opportunity to correct a knee flexion contracture if needed. Long-term results indicate that partial

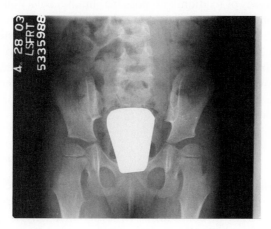

Fig. 5. Preoperative radiograph of a 4-year-old girl who has spastic diplegic cerebral palsy, bilateral coxa valga, and uncovering of the lateral one fourth of the femoral heads.

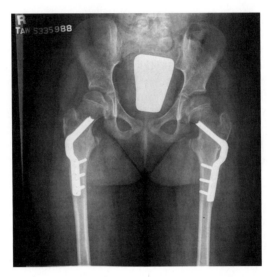

Fig. 6. Same girl as in Fig. 5 at 7 years of age after undergoing selective dorsal rhizotomy and bilateral proximal femoral rotational osteotomies and percutaneous adductor lengthenings.

recurrence of rotational deformity may occur in 0% and 33% of cases, with surgery before 10 years of age more likely to show deterioration [89,91]. Some centers avoid postoperative casting and encourage early mobilization [88]. Complications of femoral osteotomies include loss of fixation, delayed union, hardware failure, wound dehiscence or infection, and over- or under-correction [90,92].

Tibial torsion can also be surgically corrected using a tibial derotational osteotomy (Figs. 7–9). Various surgical techniques have been described, including proximal versus distal site of osteotomy, different shapes of osteotomy, various types of fixation, and possible simultaneous fibular osteotomy [86,92–94]. Complications include delayed union, cross-union, or nonunion; wound dehiscence; osteomyelitis; late fracture; distal physeal closure; and neurovascular compromise [93,94]. When combined with a split tibialis posterior tendon transfer for spastic equinovarus deformity, severe planovalgus or rigid equinovarus deformity has a higher rate of development presumably because of the increased difficulty in balancing the muscle forces across the spastic equinovarus foot [95].

Hip dysplasia

Hip dysplasia, subluxation, and dislocation are orthopedic abnormalities encountered in children who have neuromuscular disorders. Hip dysplasia refers to a spectrum of conditions of the hip that may be present at or shortly after birth, including inadequate acetabular formation, femoral head subluxation, and femoral head dislocation [96]. Hip subluxation and

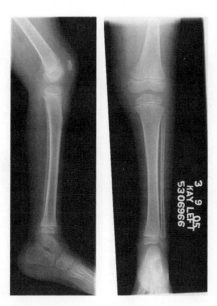

Fig. 7. Preoperative radiograph of a 5-year-old girl who has lumbar myelomeningocele and bilateral internal tibial torsion with severe intoeing.

hip dislocation have typically been defined by the hip migration percentage or Riemers' migration index, as measured on an anteroposterior radiograph. This measures the femoral head's containment within the acetabulum in the coronal plane with respect to Perkin's line [97–100] (Fig. 10). Shenton's

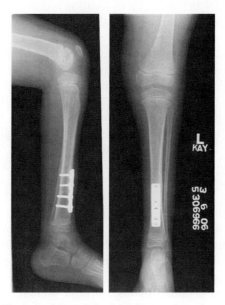

Fig. 8. Same girl as in Fig. 7 after bilateral distal tibial external rotation–producing osteotomies.

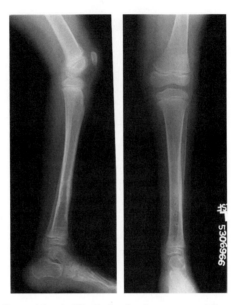

Fig. 9. Same girl as in Fig. 7 after hardware removal 2 years later.

line, which is formed by the medial aspect of the obturator foramen and the medial aspect of the femoral neck, forms an unbroken arc in the normal hip. However, in a dislocated hip, this arc will be discontinuous (see Fig. 10). Hip subluxation is usually diagnosed with a hip migration percentage of greater than 33%, although others may classify subluxation as mild when it exceeds 20% [21,99,101,102]. Hip dislocation is diagnosed when the migration percentage is greater than 100% or the femoral head is completely uncovered [102].

Other bony abnormalities, such as a shallow acetabulum, coxa valga, and femoral anteversion, are commonly associated with or contribute to femoral subluxation or dislocation. Radiographic measurements are used to evaluate these hip abnormalities. The acetabular index measures the slope of the acetabular roof compared with Hilgenreiner's line (see Fig. 10). An acetabular index of greater than 30° indicates dislocation, although accuracy of the measurement depends on patient positioning and age. Coxa valga is an increased neck–shaft angle of the femur. The neck–shaft angle of a newborn is typically 150° and typically 120° to 135°in an adult. Coxa valga in an adult is defined as an angle of greater than 135° (Fig. 11).

The most common functional impairments related to hip dysplasia include difficulty with seating, positioning, transfers, perineal hygiene, dressing, and pain [103,104]. Other potential issues include pressure sores and deformity. Seating issues are often complex because many of these children have concomitant pelvic obliquity and scoliosis.

In those who have milder disease or later presentation, the functional impairment may be less severe and occur late. For example, hip abnormalities

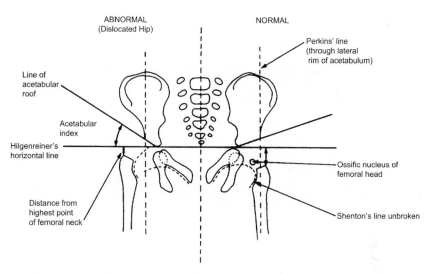

Fig. 10. Radiologic findings in congenital dislocation of the hip (*left*) compared with normal findings in a 12- to 15-month-old child (*right*). The acetabular index is increased on the dislocated side compared with normal. In an older child who has an ossified but dislocated femoral head, the migration index would be 100%. In other words, the femoral head would be found entirely lateral to the Perkin's line. Shenton's line, drawn along the medial curved edge of the femur and the inferior edge of the pubis, is broken on the dislocated side but smooth on the normal side. (*Adapted from* Magee DJ. Orthopedic physical assessment, 4th edition. Philadelphia: Saunders; 2002. p. 626; with permission.)

in children who have Charcot-Marie-Tooth disease are generally asymptomatic and may be found on radiographs obtained for other reasons. Often the hip abnormality goes undetected until adolescence or adulthood when the patient presents with a gait abnormality and pain. Pain tends to be seen in the later stages of the hip disorder when the joint may have marked subluxation or arthrodesis [105,106].

Epidemiology

In children who have no known neuromuscular disorder, the incidence of congenital hip dysplasia is 1 per 85 births with a 5:1 female-to-male ratio [107,108]. Risk factors for congenital hip dysplasia include a family history of congenital hip dysplasia, first born, female gender, and breech delivery; 25% are bilateral. When unilateral, it is four times more common in left hip [107–109].

In comparison, children who have neuromuscular disorders have an incidence of hip disorders of 8% to 82%, depending on the neuromuscular disorder, age of onset, and severity (see Table 1) [21–23,110,111]. The prevalence of hip dysplasia in cerebral palsy varies from 2% to 60%, with higher prevalence among children who are quadriplegic or nonambulatory, or have severe spasticity [110–112]. In cerebral palsy, the risk for subluxation or

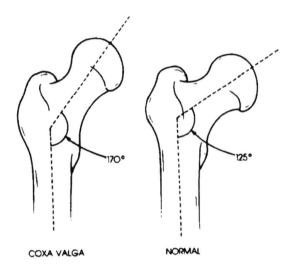

Fig. 11. Coxa valga denotes an increased neck–shaft angle compared with normal (125° in an adult). (*Adapted from* Magee DJ. Orthopedic physical assessment, 4th edition. Philadelphia: Saunders; 2002. p. 627; with permission.)

dislocation is directly related to gross motor function as measured with the Gross Motor Function Classification System (GMFCS) [113]. In children who have with spinal cord injury, the incidence of hip subluxation or dislocation is inversely related to age (ie, the older the child at injury, the lower the incidence of hip subluxation or dislocation) [21,22].

Etiology

In children who have congenital hip dysplasia without an underlying neuromuscular disorder, the most likely causes are related to intrauterine positioning, hormones, and joint laxity. In upper motor neuron disorders, such as cerebral palsy and spinal cord injury, the underlying cause of the hip disorder is a combination of muscular imbalance, spasticity, contractures, and limited ambulation. For example, muscular imbalance may be manifest through spastic hip flexors and hip adductors. This imbalance may cause asymmetric forces on the developing bony structures of the hip, resulting in deformities such as femoral anteversion, flattening of the femoral head and acetabulum, posterolateral migration of the femoral head, and flexion–adduction contractures [97,99,103,114,115]. In addition, children who have severe spasticity are often nonambulatory. The combination of a lack of ambulation and asymmetric muscle forces at the hip can exacerbate abnormalities of the femoral head and acetabulum. This results in increased forces at the lesser trochanter because of a shift in the mechanical axis of the hip with posterolateral migration of the femoral head. As the hip migration and increased lesser trochanter forces continue, subluxation, dislocation, and coxa valga may occur [111,114,116].

Similar factors occur in lower motor neuron disorders, such as spinal muscular atrophy and Charcot-Marie-Tooth disease. Global proximal weakness, limited weight-bearing, and ligamentous laxity may cause coxa valga. Trochanteric apophyseal growth may be diminished secondary to decreased weight-bearing and gluteal weakness, further promoting the coxa valga deformity [117,118]. In Charcot-Marie–Tooth disease, the proximal weakness is more subtle but may still result in a shallow acetabulum and a valgus anteverted femoral neck [106]. Children who have myopathies such as Duchenne's muscular dystrophy are often independently mobile and ambulatory during crucial times of hip development. As a result, hip disorders are less likely but still possible given the muscular imbalance. Finally, the hip dysplasia associated with congenital torticollis has an uncertain origin. However, the conditions causing the development of the torticollis may participate in the development of hip dysplasia [119].

Natural history of hip dysplasia

In congenital hip dysplasia, congruent reduction achieved before 4 years of age typically results in normal hip development [120]. Evidence shows that proper hip development requires the femoral head to be centralized in the acetabulum by or around 5 years of age [121–123].

In a study of children who had quadriplegic cerebral palsy who did not walk, the mean hip migration index was 12% per year. In ambulatory children, the hip migration index was 2% per year. Ambulatory status and age were found to be the most influential factors on rate of progression of hip migration, and therefore young, nonambulatory children tend to have more rapid progression of hip migration [124].

Pelvic obliquity may coexist with hip subluxation, hip dislocation, scoliosis, and "wind-swept" hips (adduction of one hip and abduction of the other hip). The relationship between pelvic obliquity and hip dysplasia is controversial [96,121,125–128]. Suprapelvic obliquity refers to obliquity secondary to scoliosis, whereas infrapelvic obliquity refers to imbalance below the pelvis. One study of children who had spastic cerebral palsy found that the development of hip dysplasia was more related to infrapelvic obliquity than suprapelvic obliquity. Infrapelvic obliquity was noted to precede suprapelvic obliquity, and hip subluxation and dislocation almost always occurred on the high side [129].

Evaluation

Key elements of the history related to hip dysplasia include intrauterine abnormalities such as oligohydramnios; birth difficulties such as breech birth; and a family history of hip disorders in children or young adults. A review of symptoms, including the presence of pain, decreased sitting tolerance, autonomic dysreflexia, and skin ulcers, is critical [130,131]. A hip physical examination for dysplasia includes an evaluation of the presence of an asymmetry of fat folds of the thigh and buttocks; a Trendelenburg's sign; limitations of passive range of motion in all directions, including asymmetry; "popping," or pain. Hip flexion contractures are evaluated using the Thomas test and rectus tightness using the Ely test. Hip adduction contractures may be assessed with the hip and knee in extension (gracilis stretch) and flexion. Hip rotation is best assessed with the child prone. An apparent leg length discrepancy may be evaluated using the Galeazzi sign (Fig. 12), for which the child lies supine with knees and hips flexed. If the knees are not at the same height, the low side may be posteriorly subluxed or dislocated. One may also evaluate for a *telescoping sign* (Fig. 13) in which the child is again placed supine with hips and knees flexed, and the femur is pushed posteriorly toward the table and lifted up. A normal hip will show little motion, but a dislocated hip will reveal an excessive telescoping or pistoning movement.

Special maneuvers, such as the Ortolani and Barlow tests, are used in infants (Fig. 14). With the child calm and pelvis stable, the Ortolani test is performed by first flexing the knee and hip. The thigh is then abducted while applying slight traction to the distal thigh and slight anterior pressure against the trochanters. If the hip is dislocated before starting the maneuver, one may palpate a relocation "clunk." The Barlow test continues from this position. The hip is then adducted with a slight compressive force backward and outward on the inner thigh while palpating for a "clunk."

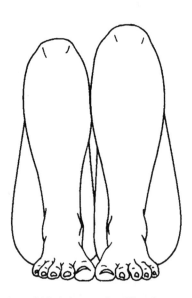

Fig. 12. The Galeazzi sign is useful in infants and toddlers for assessing unilateral hip dislocation or dysplasia. (*Adapted from* Magee DJ. Orthopedic physical assessment, 4th edition. Philadelphia: Saunders; 2002. p. 627; with permission.)

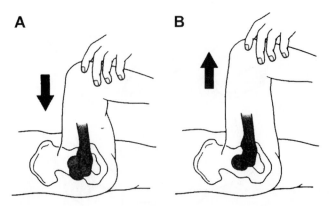

Fig. 13. Telescoping of the hip occurs if the hip is not fixed in the acetabulum. (*Adapted from* Magee DJ. Orthopedic physical assessment, 4th edition. Philadelphia: Saunders; 2002. p. 629; with permission.)

Anteroposterior radiographs of the pelvis with legs extended may show subluxation, dislocation, and lateral notching of the femoral head (Fig. 15). The lateral notching has been hypothesized to be caused by chronic pressure from ligamentum teres, the joint capsule, the reflected portion of the rectus femoris, and the hip abductor musculature, but was recently found to be most likely caused by a spastic gluteus minimus [132]. A systematic literature review evaluating the evidence on hip surveillance in children who have cerebral palsy concluded that all children who have bilateral cerebral palsy should have a radiograph of the hips at age 30 months or sooner if clinically suspicious. Children who have a migration index greater than 33% or acetabular index greater than 30° are most likely to require further treatment of their hips, particularly if noted by 30 months of age [110]. Others recommend that children who have more severe neuromuscular disorders, such as quadriplegic cerebral palsy, undergo a radiograph of the pelvis at 1 year of age and yearly thereafter until the natural history has been established. Children who have spastic diplegia should begin screening at 2 to 3 years of age, with subsequent radiographs every 2 to 3 years [124]. In infants who have Charcot-Marie-Tooth type 1, a screening ultrasound is recommended. In Charcot-Marie-Tooth type 2, screening with pelvis radiographs at least every 2 years is recommended [106].

In newborns, ultrasound is the recommended imaging modality if a hip abnormality is suspected based on history or physical examination, because ultrasound can image cartilage. Because the femoral heads do not ossify until 3 to 6 months of age, radiographs may not completely show the femoral–acetabular relationship [107]. Repeat ultrasound imaging is recommended because false-positive findings are not uncommon in newborns.

Other imaging modalities, such as CT or MRI, may be considered in selected cases. Three-dimensional CT may provide additional detail about the femoral head and acetabular relationship, thus aiding in surgical

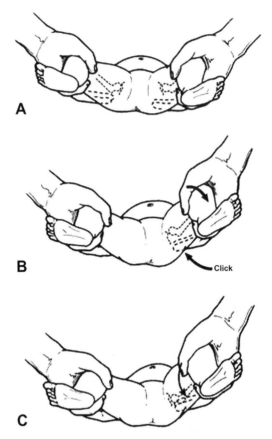

Fig. 14. Ortolani's sign and Barlow's test. (*A*) In the newborn, the two hips can be equally flexed, abducted, and laterally rotated without producing a "click." (*B*) Ortolani's sign or first part of Barlow's test. (*C*) Second part of Barlow's test. (*Adapted from* Magee DJ. Orthopedic physical assessment, 4th edition. Philadelphia: Saunders; 2002. p. 648; with permission.)

planning. CT, for example, may provide more comprehensive evaluation of the location of acetabular dysplasia. The most common location of acetabular dysplasia is posterior, but abnormalities have been noted in other locations, including anterior, midsuperior, anterosuperior, posterosuperior, and global [133]. Although used infrequently, MRI may be useful for evaluating the hip with an unossified femoral head that has been resistant to conservative treatment and may not be otherwise adequately imaged for presurgical planning [134].

Nonoperative treatment for hip dysplasia

A physical therapy program performed by therapists and caregivers, with daily focus on stretching of tight muscles, positioning, weight-bearing, and orthotic devices is essential. Maintaining flexibility of two joint muscles,

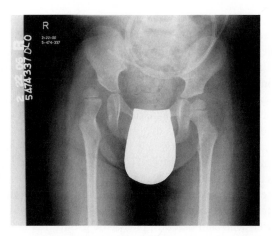

Fig. 15. Radiographs of a 5-year-old boy who has linear sebaceous nevus syndrome and right hemiplegia. Bilateral coxa valga, right greater than left. Superolateral subluxation of the right femoral head, which is covered less than 10% by the shallow acetabulum. Less than one fourth uncovering of the left femoral head.

such as the gastrocnemius, hamstrings, gracilis, and rectus femoris, is important. Standing or walking with or without orthoses has been shown to be crucial in delaying or preventing hip subluxation or dislocation in children who have upper and lower motor neuron disorders [25,123].

Nonoperative treatment approaches for developmental hip dysplasia include orthotics such as the Pavlik harness, Frejka pillow, Craig splint, or Van Rosen splint. The Pavlik harness is most commonly used [96]. These orthoses are intended to provide a prolonged stretch to hypertonic or tight hip adductors and promote correct acetabular development and spontaneous reduction of subluxed or dislocated hips. However, use of abduction bracing is contraindicated in patients who have lower motor neuron disorders, ligamentous laxity (Ehlers-Danlos syndrome), or fixed deformities (arthrogryposis) [106,135].

Other methods of postural management have been evaluated, although studies are small and use different postural devices. Postural devices include systems such as prone and supine lying supports, standing frames, and wheel chair seating systems, which all attempt to keep the hips in an abducted position. The amount of time the specific device is used depends on the severity of the hip migration, type of device used, and child's tolerance. Some systems are recommended for up to 24-hour use. Studies have shown benefit when these devices are worn as intended [130,136,137].

Spasticity is believed to be a contributor to hip subluxation and dislocation in children who have cerebral palsy. Therefore, aggressive spasticity treatment has been speculated to reduce the progression of spastic hip disease. The effects of intrathecal baclofen on spasticity reduction are well known. One prospective, open-label, multicenter case series has been published on intrathecal baclofen and hip dysplasia in 33 children. The participants ranged from 4 to 31 years of age and included those who had paraplegic, tetraplegic, and diplegic cerebral palsy; most were nonambulatory. They were followed up for 1 year. The hip migration percentage stabilized or decreased in more than 90% of participants, with a trend toward greater improvement in younger participants. No controls were included, and more than two thirds of participants experienced at least one adverse event post-implant, including some serious drug-related events [138].

The effect of a single botulinum A injection to hip adductors was evaluated in one small retrospective study. Children who had an initial migration percentage greater than 30% who were younger than 24 months at injection were most likely to exhibit stabilization or improvement in the migration percentage during the 6-month follow-up [139]. In a randomized prospective study of children who had cerebral palsy, the group treated with botulinum A and a variable hip abductor brace required soft tissue surgery for hip adductor muscles less often than a control group who underwent standard physical therapy only. However, longer-term outcomes are not yet available [140]. Although more research is needed, a combination of botulinum A, hip abduction orthoses, and physical therapy starting in children younger than 24 months may prevent or delay hip disorders. In children who had cerebral palsy who underwent dorsal rhizotomies, the subsequent frequency of hip subluxation or dislocation was most often stable or reduced [141].

Operative treatment

The goal of operative intervention for hip dysplasia is to maintain mobile, located hips so that sitting balance, ambulatory ability, and comfort are enhanced. Operative interventions include soft tissue lengthening and hip reconstruction using femoral osteotomy with or without pelvic osteotomy. Salvage procedures are available for patients who have deformity of the femoral head, breakdown of articular cartilage, and established dislocation that cannot be repaired. In neuromuscular hip dysplasia, surgical intervention may be necessary when hip deformity or disability has progressed despite maximal conservative intervention. The timing of surgical intervention and type of intervention have been debated. However, hips with a migration percentage greater than 50% frequently require surgical intervention because of the risk for further progression and dislocation [124,142]. In addition, hips with greater than 70% of the femoral head uncovered preoperatively have a higher incidence of instability postoperatively [143].

Soft tissue procedures are often recommended as a prophylactic measure against the development of bony deformity. In patients who do not have bony deformity, these procedures may play a role in stabilizing the hip. Procedures include iliopsoas, hamstring, and adductor release or lengthening. A review of the evidence for hip adductor release used to prevent progressive hip subluxation in children who had cerebral palsy was recently published. Despite difficulties related to study design, a few observations were made. Radiographic improvement after adductor release was seen in approximately 50% of hips. However, the clinical significance and correlation to improvement of pain, function, or activities of daily living has not been systematically evaluated. Children who have a smaller preoperative hip migration index have a decreased incidence of postoperative hip resubluxation or progression of migration index. Specifically, preoperative migration percentages of less than 30% to 40% were associated with successful outcomes in 75% to 90% of hips. Reported complications were few, although unilateral hip adductor release was often noted to have an adverse effect on the contralateral hip [144].

When bony abnormalities such as femoral torsion, coxa valga, and deformity of the acetabulum have occurred, bony procedures may be necessary and are often performed in conjunction with soft tissue releases. In patients who have no marked deformity of the acetabulum, surgical emphasis is placed on correcting femoral abnormalities. Possible interventions include derotational osteotomy of the femur, correction of the neck–shaft angle (coxa valga), and shortening of the femur to decrease muscle forces across the hip [111].

In patients who have coexisting acetabular deficiency, pelvic osteotomy may be required. The Pemberton osteotomy or acetabuloplasty (Figs. 16 and 17) is indicated if a deficiency of the anterior and superolateral walls of acetabulum is present. The Salter pelvic innominate procedure is used for anterolateral acetabular deficiency. The Dega osteotomy is typically indicated for posterior hip dislocations. The modified Dega adds femoral or intertrochanteric osteotomies or open hip reduction (Figs. 18, 19). The

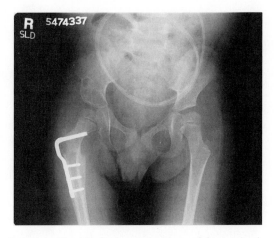

Fig. 16. Same patient as in Fig. 15 who has undergone a right proximal varus and external rotation–producing osteotomy and Pemberton periacetabular osteotomy with bone graft from the iliac crest.

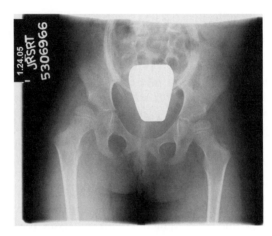

Fig. 17. Four-year-old girl who has lumbar myelomeningocele. Lateral uncovering of 50% of the right femoral head by the acetabulum and one fourth uncovering of the left femoral head.

San Diego procedure is used for anteroposterior acetabular deficiency and includes a femoral osteotomy and soft tissue releases. The Bernese (Ganz) periacetabular osteotomy may be performed in adolescents and adults who have dysplastic hips that require correction of congruency and containment to the femoral head. This procedure may be combined with a proximal femoral osteotomy to provide uninvolved acetabular and proximal femoral weight-bearing surfaces. The Chiari procedure is typically a salvage procedure that places the femoral head under a surface of cancellous bone rather than articular cartilage and is recommended in older children who have

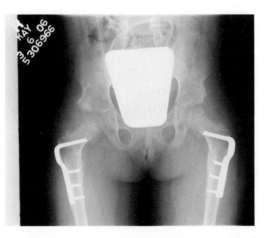

Fig. 18. Same girl as in Fig. 17 after undergoing right open hip reduction with capsulorrhaphy, bilateral Dega pelvic osteotomies, and bilateral proximal femoral varus and external rotation–producing osteotomies.

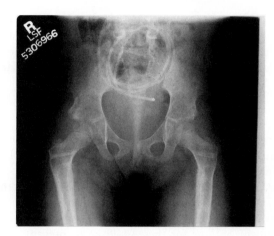

Fig. 19. Same girl as in Fig. 18 two years after hardware removed.

severe dysplasia and possibly subluxation when no other reconstructive options are available. A Shelf salvage procedure uses a bone graft for added support to the femoral head. The merits and outcomes of these various procedures are debated [102,103,128,142,143,145–149].

In nonambulatory children who have minimal symptoms or seating difficulties, operative treatment of hip subluxation or dislocation is controversial. Operative treatment options are similar for children who have upper and lower motor neuron disorders with a few exceptions. For individuals who have Charcot-Marie-Tooth disease and hip dysplasia, the acetabular deficiency has been recommended to be repaired first, because a primary femoral derotational osteotomy in the setting of weak hip abductors may exacerbate a Trendelenburg's gait. If femoral derotational osteotomy is subsequently needed, the surgeon is suggested to proceed with internal fixation and early mobilization, because spica casts may exacerbate hip weakness from prolonged immobilization [106]. In children who have spinal muscular atrophy, a high frequency of resubluxation after surgical intervention has been reported [117,118,150]. Therefore, surgical intervention for subluxed or dislocated hips in children who have intermediate spinal muscular atrophy is not generally recommended. However, if surgical intervention is believed necessary, a single-stage combined procedure of appropriate soft tissue release and bony reconstruction is pursued [25,117,118,150]. A review of hip disorders in children who have spinal cord injury noted that operative treatment should include release of soft tissue contractures and appropriate bony interventions with muscle transfers in a select group of patients. Postoperatively, a hip abduction orthosis rather than casting is recommended to reduce risk for skin breakdown [130]. In congenital hip dysplasia, surgical correction usually involves closed reduction with casting. This procedure should be considered when a Pavlik harness trial of 6 to 12 weeks has failed or the patient is older than 6 months [134]. If closed reduction is not possible or a child has a more advanced deformity, open reduction may be considered. Open reduction may combine soft tissue release and femoral shortening with varus derotational osteotomy, with or without acetabular osteotomy.

Summary

A wide variety of neuromuscular diseases affect children. Despite the vastly different primary pathophysiologic mechanisms of these disorders, certain secondary musculoskeletal complications are shared. Scoliosis, bony rotational deformities, and hip dysplasia are some of the most common sequelae in children. Care providers must recognize the musculoskeletal abnormalities and understand the natural history and nonoperative and operative treatment options for these children to prevent progression and functional loss.

References

[1] Giannini S, Faldini C, Pagkrati S, et al. Surgical treatment of neck hyperextension in Duchenne muscular dystrophy by posterior interspinous fusion. Spine 2006;31:1805–9.
[2] Chu WC, Li AM, Ng BK, et al. Dynamic magnetic resonance imaging in assessing lung volumes, chest wall, and diaphragm motions in adolescent idiopathic scoliosis versus normal controls. Spine 2006;31:2243–9.
[3] Block AJ, Wexler J, McDonnell EJ. Cardiopulmonary failure of the hunchback. A possible therapeutic approach. JAMA 1970;212:1520–2.
[4] Bunnell WP. The natural history of idiopathic scoliosis. Clin Orthop Relat Res 1988;20–5.
[5] Rosenthal RK, Levine DB, McCarver CL. The occurrence of scoliosis in cerebral palsy. Dev Med Child Neurol 1974;16:664–7.
[6] Madigan RR, Wallace SL. Scoliosis in the institutionalized cerebral palsy population. Spine 1981;6:583–90.
[7] Muller EB, Nordwall A. Prevalence of scoliosis in children with myelomeningocele in western Sweden. Spine 1992;17:1097–102.
[8] Kinali M, Messina S, Mercuri E, et al. Management of scoliosis in Duchenne muscular dystrophy: a large 10-year retrospective study. Dev Med Child Neurol 2006;48:513–8.
[9] Granata C, Merlini L, Cervellati S, et al. Long-term results of spine surgery in Duchenne muscular dystrophy. Neuromuscul Disord 1996;6:61–8.
[10] Mayfield JK, Erkkila JC, Winter RB. Spine deformity subsequent to acquired childhood spinal cord injury. J Bone Joint Surg Am 1981;63:1401–11.
[11] Hensinger R. Spinal deformity associated with heritable neurological conditions: spinal muscular atrophy, Friedreich's ataxia, familial dysautonomia and Charcot-Marie-Tooth disease. J Bone Joint Surg Am 1976;58:13–24.
[12] Evans GA, Drennan JC, Russman BS. Functional classification and orthopaedic management of spinal muscular atrophy. J Bone Joint Surg Br 1981;63:516–22.
[13] Russman BS. Spinal muscular atrophy. Muscle Nerve 1983;6:179–81.
[14] Schwentker EP, Gibson DA. The orthopaedic aspects of spinal muscular atrophy. J Bone Joint Surg Am 1976;58:32–8.
[15] Lonstein JE, Beck K. Hip dislocation and subluxation in cerebral palsy. J Pediatr Orthop 1986;6:521–6.

[16] Cooke PH, Cole WG, Carey RP. Dislocation of the hip in cerebral palsy. Natural history and predictability. J Bone Joint Surg Br 1989;71:441–6.

[17] Hagglund G, Andersson S, Duppe H, et al. Prevention of dislocation of the hip in children with cerebral palsy. The first ten years of a population-based prevention programme. J Bone Joint Surg Br 2005;87:95–101.

[18] Mathews SS, Jones MH, Sperling SC. Hip derangements seen in cerebral palsied children. Am J Phys Med 1953;32:213–21.

[19] Broughton NS, Menelaus MB, Cole WG, et al. The natural history of hip deformity in myelomeningocele. J Bone Joint Surg Br 1993;75:760–3.

[20] Chan K. Hip subluxation and dislocation in Duchenne muscular dystrophy. J Pediatr Orthop B 2001;10:219–25.

[21] McCarthy JJ, Chafetz RS, Betz RR, et al. Incidence and degree of hip subluxation/dislocation in children with spinal cord injury. J Spinal Cord Med 2004;27(Suppl 1):S80–3.

[22] Vogel LC, Lubicky JP. Ambulation in children and adolescents with spinal cord injuries. J Pediatr Orthop 1995;15:510–6.

[23] Rink P, Miller F. Hip instability in spinal cord injury patients. J Pediatr Orthop 1990;10: 583–7.

[24] Walker JL, Nelson KR, Heavilon JA, et al. Hip abnormalities in children with Charcot-Marie-Tooth disease. J Pediatr Orthop 1994;14:54–9.

[25] Granata C, Magni E, Merlini L, et al. Hip dislocation in spinal muscular atrophy. Chir Organi Mov 1990;75:177–84.

[26] Deacon P, Dickson RA. Vertebral shape in the median sagittal plane in idiopathic thoracic scoliosis. A study of true lateral radiographs in 150 patients. Orthopedics 1987;10:893–5.

[27] Johnson MB, Goldstein L, Thomas SS, et al. Spinal deformity after selective dorsal rhizotomy in ambulatory patients with cerebral palsy. J Pediatr Orthop 1987;24:529–36.

[28] Steinbok P, Hicdonmez T, Sawatzky B, et al. Spinal deformities after selective dorsal rhizotomy for spastic cerebral palsy. J Neurosurg 2005;102:363–73.

[29] Giampietro PF, Blank RD, Raggio CL, et al. Congenital and idiopathic scoliosis: clinical and genetic aspects. Clin Med Res 2003;1:125–36.

[30] Burwell RG, Freeman BJ, Dangerfield PH, et al. Etiologic theories of idiopathic scoliosis: neurodevelopmental concept of maturational delay of the CNS body schema ("body-in-the-brain"). Stud Health Technol Inform 2006;123:72–9.

[31] Stokes I. Hueter-Volkmann effect, vol. 14. Philadelphia: Hanley & Belfus, Inc.; 2000. p. 349–57.

[32] Hawes MC, O'Brien JP. The transformation of spinal curvature into spinal deformity: pathological processes and implications for treatment. Scoliosis 2006;1:3.

[33] Berven S, Bradford DS. Neuromuscular scoliosis: causes of deformity and principles for evaluation and management. Semin Neurol 2002;22:167–78.

[34] Haberl H, Tallen G, Michael T, et al. Surgical aspects and outcome of delayed tethered cord release. Zentralbl Neurochir 2004;65:161–7.

[35] Sarwark JF, Weber DT, Gabrieli AP, et al. Tethered cord syndrome in low motor level children with myelomeningocele. Pediatr Neurosurg 1996;25:295–301.

[36] Fribourg D, Delgado E. Occult spinal cord abnormalities in children referred for orthopedic complaints. Am J Orthop 2004;33:18–25.

[37] Loder RT, Spiegel D, Gutknecht S. The assessment of intraobserver and interobserver error in the measurement of noncongenital scoliosis in children < or = years of age. Spine 2004; 29:2548–53.

[38] Kouwenhoven JW, Van Ommeren PM, Pruijs HE, et al. Spinal decompensation in neuromuscular disease. Spine 2006;31:E188–91.

[39] Hamzaoglu A, Talu U, Tezer M, et al. Assessment of curve flexibility in adolescent idiopathic scoliosis. Spine 2005;30:1637–42.

[40] Hawes MC. The use of exercises in the treatment of scoliosis: an evidence-based critical review of the literature. Pediatr Rehabil 2003;6:171–82.

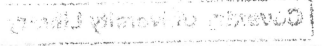

[41] Maruyama T, Kitagawa T, Takeshita K, et al. Conservative treatment for adolescent idiopathic scoliosis: can it reduce the incidence of surgical treatment? Pediatr Rehabil 2003;6: 215–9.

[42] Morningstar MW, Woggon D, Lawrence G. Scoliosis treatment using a combination of manipulative and rehabilitative therapy: a retrospective case series. BMC Musculoskelet Disord 2004;5:32.

[43] Weiss HR. Rehabilitation of adolescent patients with scoliosis—what do we know? A review of the literature. Pediatr Rehabil 2003;6:183–94.

[44] Olafsson Y, Saraste H, Al-Dabbagh Z. Brace treatment in neuromuscular spine deformity. J Pediatr Orthop 1999;19:376–9.

[45] Muller EB, Nordwall A. Brace treatment of scoliosis in children with myelomeningocele. Spine 1994;19:151–5.

[46] Miller A, Temple T, Miller F. Impact of orthoses on the rate of scoliosis progression in children with cerebral palsy. J Pediatr Orthop 1996;16:332–5.

[47] Kilmer DD. The role of exercise in neuromuscular disease. Phys Med Rehabil Clin N Am 1998;9:115–25.

[48] Ansved T. Muscle training in muscular dystrophies. Acta Physiol Scand 2001;171:359–66.

[49] Ansved T. Muscular dystrophies: influence of physical conditioning on the disease evolution. Curr Opin Clin Nutr Metab Care 2003;6:435–9.

[50] Wright NC, Kilmer DD, McCrory MA, et al. Aerobic walking in slowly progressive neuromuscular disease: effect of a 12-week program. Arch Phys Med Rehabil 1996;77:64–9.

[51] Rodgers WB, Frim DM, Emans JB. Surgery of the spine in myelodysplasia. An overview. Clin Orthop Relat Res 1997;19–35.

[52] Bayar B, Uygur F, Bayar K, et al. The short -term effects of an exercise programme as an adjunct to an orthosis in neuromuscular scoliosis. Prosthet Orthot Int 2004;28:273–7.

[53] Leopando MT, Moussavi Z, Holbrow J, et al. Effect of a Soft Boston Orthosis on pulmonary mechanics in severe cerebral palsy. Pediatr Pulmonol 1999;28:53–8.

[54] Muntoni F, Bushby K, Manzur AY. Muscular Dystrophy Campaign Funded Workshop on Management of Scoliosis in Duchenne Muscular Dystrophy 24 January 2005, London, UK. Neuromuscul Disord 2006;16:210–9.

[55] Yilmaz O, Karaduman A, Topalolu H. Prednisolone therapy in Duchenne muscular dystrophy prolongs ambulation and prevents scoliosis. Eur J Neurol 2004;11:541–4.

[56] Balaban B, Matthews DJ, Clayton GH, et al. Corticosteroid treatment and functional improvement in Duchenne muscular dystrophy: long-term effect. Am J Phys Med Rehabil 2005;84:843–50.

[57] Rodillo EB, Fernandez-Bermejo E, Heckmatt JZ, et al. Prevention of rapidly progressive scoliosis in Duchenne muscular dystrophy by prolongation of walking with orthoses. J Child Neurol 1988;3:269–74.

[58] Alman BA, Raza SN, Biggar WD. Steroid treatment and the development of scoliosis in males with Duchenne muscular dystrophy. J Bone Joint Surg Am 2004;86:519–24.

[59] Larsson EL, Aaro SI, Normelli HC, et al. Long-term follow-up of functioning after spinal surgery in patients with neuromuscular scoliosis. Spine 2005;30:2145–52.

[60] Crawford JR, Izatt MT, Adam CJ, et al. A prospective assessment of SRS-24 scores after endoscopic anterior instrumentation for scoliosis. Spine 2006;31:E817–22.

[61] Askin GN, Hallett R, Hare N, et al. The outcome of scoliosis surgery in the severely physically handicapped child. An objective and subjective assessment. Spine 1997;22:44–50.

[62] Miller F, Moseley CF, Koreska J. Spinal fusion in Duchenne muscular dystrophy. Dev Med Child Neurol 1992;34:775–86.

[63] Kennedy JD, Staples AJ, Brook PD, et al. Effect of spinal surgery on lung function in Duchenne muscular dystrophy. Thorax 1995;50:1173–8.

[64] Takeshita K, Lenke LG, Bridwell KH, et al. Analysis of patients with nonambulatory neuromuscular scoliosis surgically treated to the pelvis with intraoperative halo-femoral traction. Spine 2006;31:2381–5.

[65] Sengupta DK, Mehdian SH, McConnell JR, et al. Pelvic or lumbar fixation for the surgical management of scoliosis in Duchenne muscular dystrophy. Spine 2002;27:2072–9.

[66] Akbarnia BA, Marks DS, Boachie-Adjei O, et al. Dual growing rod technique for the treatment of progressive early-onset scoliosis: a multicenter study. Spine 2005;30:S46–57.

[67] Cervellati S, Bettini N, Moscato M, et al. Surgical treatment of spinal deformities in Duchenne muscular dystrophy: a long term follow-up study. Eur Spine J 2004;13: 441–8.

[68] Murphy NA, Firth S, Jorgensen T, et al. Spinal surgery in children with idiopathic and neuromuscular scoliosis. What's the difference? J Pediatr Orthop 2006;26:216–20.

[69] Gaine WJ, Lim J, Stephenson W, et al. Progression of scoliosis after spinal fusion in Duchenne's muscular dystrophy. J Bone Joint Surg Br 2004;86:550–5.

[70] Tsirikos AI, Chang WN, Dabney KW, et al. Life expectancy in pediatric patients with cerebral palsy and neuromuscular scoliosis who underwent spinal fusion. Dev Med Child Neurol 2003;45:677–82.

[71] Wazeka AN, DiMaio MF, Boachie-Adjei O. Outcome of pediatric patients with severe restrictive lung disease following reconstructive spine surgery. Spine 2004;29:528–34.

[72] Gill I, Eagle M, Mehta JS, et al. Correction of neuromuscular scoliosis in patients with pre-existing respiratory failure. Spine 2006;31:2478–83.

[73] Almenrader N, Patel D. Spinal fusion surgery in children with non-idiopathic scoliosis: is there a need for routine postoperative ventilation? Br J Anaesth 2006;97:851–7.

[74] Gage JR. Gait analysis. An essential tool in the treatment of cerebral palsy. Clin Orthop Relat Res 1993;126–34.

[75] Gage JR, DeLuca PA, Renshaw TS. Gait analysis: principle and applications with emphasis on its use in cerebral palsy. Instr Course Lect 1996;45:491–507.

[76] Eckhoff DG, Kramer RC, Alongi CA, et al. Femoral anteversion and arthritis of the knee. J Pediatr Orthop 1994;14:608–10.

[77] Eckhoff DG, Montgomery WK, Kilcoyne RF, et al. Femoral morphometry and anterior knee pain. Clin Orthop Relat Res 1994;64–8.

[78] Halpern AA, Tanner J, Rinsky L. Does persistent fetal femoral anteversion contribute to osteoarthritis?: a preliminary report. Clin Orthop Relat Res 1979;213–6.

[79] Yagi T. Tibial torsion in patients with medial-type osteoarthrotic knees. Clin Orthop Relat Res 1994;52–6.

[80] Rethlefsen SA, Healy BS, Wren TA, et al. Causes of intoeing gait in children with cerebral palsy. J Bone Joint Surg Am 2006;88:2175–80.

[81] O'Sullivan R, Walsh M, Hewart P, et al. Factors associated with internal hip rotation gait in patients with cerebral palsy. J Pediatr Orthop 2006;26:537–41.

[82] Arnold AS, Delp SL. Rotational moment arms of the medial hamstrings and adductors vary with femoral geometry and limb position: implications for the treatment of internally rotated gait. J Biomech 2001;34:437–47.

[83] Magee D. Orthopedic physical assessment. 4th edition. Philadelphia: Saunders; 2002.

[84] Bobroff ED, Chambers HG, Sartoris DJ, et al. Femoral anteversion and neck-shaft angle in children with cerebral palsy. Clin Orthop Relat Res 1999;194–204.

[85] Kristiansen LP, Gunderson RB, Steen H, et al. The normal development of tibial torsion. Skeletal Radiol 2001;30:519–22.

[86] Fraser RK, Menelaus MB. The management of tibial torsion in patients with spina bifida. J Bone Joint Surg Br 1993;75:495–7.

[87] Desloovere K, Molenaers G, De Cat J, et al. Motor function following multilevel botulinum toxin type A treatment in children with cerebral palsy. Dev Med Child Neurol 2007;49: 56–61.

[88] Pirpiris M, Trivett A, Baker R, et al. Femoral derotation osteotomy in spastic diplegia. Proximal or distal? J Bone Joint Surg Br 2003;85:265–72.

[89] Ounpuu S, DeLuca P, Davis R, et al. Long-term effects of femoral derotation osteotomies: an evaluation using three-dimensional gait analysis. J Pediatr Orthop 2002;22:139–45.

[90] Kay RM, Rethlefsen SA, Hale JM, et al. Comparison of proximal and distal rotational femoral osteotomy in children with cerebral palsy. J Pediatr Orthop 2003;23:150–4.

[91] Kim H, Aiona M, Sussman M. Recurrence after femoral derotational osteotomy in cerebral palsy. J Pediatr Orthop 2005;25:739–43.

[92] Stefko RM, de Swart RJ, Dodgin DA, et al. Kinematic and kinetic analysis of distal derotational osteotomy of the leg in children with cerebral palsy. J Pediatr Orthop 1998;18:81–7.

[93] Ryan DD, Rethlefsen SA, Skaggs DL, et al. Results of tibial rotational osteotomy without concomitant fibular osteotomy in children with cerebral palsy. J Pediatr Orthop 2005;25:84–8.

[94] Dodgin DA, De Swart RJ, Stefko RM, et al. Distal tibial/fibular derotation osteotomy for correction of tibial torsion: review of technique and results in 63 cases. J Pediatr Orthop 1998;18:95–101.

[95] Liggio FJ, Kruse R. Split tibialis posterior tendon transfer with concomitant distal tibial derotational osteotomy in children with cerebral palsy. J Pediatr Orthop 2001;21:95–101.

[96] Witt C. Detecting developmental dysplasia of the hip. Advances in Neonatal Care 2003;3:65–75.

[97] Beals RK. Developmental changes in the femur and acetabulum in spastic paraplegia and diplegia. Dev Med Child Neurol 1969;11:303–13.

[98] Perkins G. Signs by which to diagnose congenital dislocation of the hip. 1928. Clin Orthop Relat Res 1992;3–5.

[99] Reimers J. The stability of the hip in children. A radiological study of the results of muscle surgery in cerebral palsy. Acta Orthop Scand Suppl 1980;184:1–100.

[100] Snyder CR. Legg-Perthes disease in the young hip—does it necessarily do well? J Bone Joint Surg Am 1975;57:751–9.

[101] Cooperman DR, Bartucci E, Dietrick E, et al. Hip dislocation in spastic cerebral palsy: long-term consequences. J Pediatr Orthop 1987;7:268–76.

[102] Heckman JD. Campbell's operative orthopaedics. J Bone Joint Surg Am 2003;85:1414.

[103] Samilson RL, Tsou P, Aamoth G, et al. Dislocation and subluxation of the hip in cerebral palsy. Pathogenesis, natural history and management. J Bone Joint Surg Am 1972;54:863–73.

[104] Letts M, Shapiro L, Mulder K, et al. The windblown hip syndrome in total body cerebral palsy. J Pediatr Orthop 1984;4:55–62.

[105] McGann R, Gurd A. The association between Charcot-Marie-Tooth disease and developmental dysplasia of the hip. Orthopedics 2002;25:337–9.

[106] Chan G, Bowen JR, Kumar SJ. Evaluation and treatment of hip dysplasia in Charcot-Marie-Tooth disease. Orthop Clin North Am 2006;37:203–9.

[107] Cady RB. Developmental dysplasia of the hip: definition, recognition, and prevention of late sequelae. Pediatr Ann 2006;35:92–101.

[108] Aronsson DD, Goldberg MJ, Kling TF Jr, et al. Developmental dysplasia of the hip [erratum appears in Pediatrics 1994 Oct;94(4 Pt 1):470]. Pediatrics 1994;94:201–8.

[109] Rosendahl K, Markestad T, Lie RT. Developmental dysplasia of the hip: prevalence based on ultrasound diagnosis. Pediatr Radiol 1996;26:635–9.

[110] Gordon GS, Simkiss DE. A systematic review of the evidence for hip surveillance in children with cerebral palsy. J Bone Joint Surg Br 2006;88:1492–6.

[111] Spiegel DA, Flynn JM. Evaluation and treatment of hip dysplasia in cerebral palsy. Orthop Clin North Am 2006;37:185–96.

[112] Morton RE, Scott B, McClelland V, et al. Dislocation of the hips in children with bilateral spastic cerebral palsy, 1985-2000. Dev Med Child Neurol 2006;48:555–8.

[113] Soo B, Howard JJ, Boyd RN, et al. Hip displacement in cerebral palsy. J Bone Joint Surg Am 2006;88:121–9.

[114] Moreau M, Drummond DS, Rogala E, et al. Natural history of the dislocated hip in spastic cerebral palsy. Dev Med Child Neurol 1979;21:749–53.

[115] Wheeler ME, Weinstein SL. Adductor tenotomy-obturator neurectomy. J Pediatr Orthop 1984;4:48–51.

[116] Gamble JG, Rinsky LA, Bleck EE. Established hip dislocations in children with cerebral palsy. Clin Orthop Relat Res 1990;90–9.

[117] Sporer SM, Smith BG. Hip dislocation in patients with spinal muscular atrophy. J Pediatr Orthop 2003;23:10–4.

[118] Zenios M, Sampath J, Cole C, et al. Operative treatment for hip subluxation in spinal muscular atrophy. J Bone Joint Surg Br 2005;87:1541–4.

[119] von Heideken J, Green DW, Burke SW, et al. The relationship between developmental dysplasia of the hip and congenital muscular torticollis. J Pediatr Orthop 2006;26:805–8.

[120] Roger M. Lyon: pediatric orthopedic radiology. In: Ozonoff MB, editor. Philadelphia: W.B. Saunders Co.; 1992. p. 803.

[121] Kalen V, Bleck EE. Prevention of spastic paralytic dislocation of the hip. Dev Med Child Neurol 1985;27:17–24.

[122] Harris NH. Acetabular growth potential in congenital dislocation of the hip and some factors upon which it may depend. Clin Orthop Relat Res 1976;99–106.

[123] Scrutton D, Baird G, Smeeton N. Hip dysplasia in bilateral cerebral palsy: incidence and natural history in children aged 18 months to 5 years. Dev Med Child Neurol 2001;43:586–600.

[124] Terjesen T. Development of the hip joints in unoperated children with cerebral palsy: a radiographic study of 76 patients. Acta Orthop 2006;77:125–31.

[125] Bleck EE. The hip in cerebral palsy. Orthop Clin North Am 1980;11:79–104.

[126] Hoffer MM. Management of the hip in cerebral palsy. J Bone Joint Surg Am 1986;68:629–31.

[127] Samilson RL. Orthopedic surgery of the hips and spine in retarded cerebral palsy patients. Orthop Clin North Am 1981;12:83–90.

[128] Hoffer MM, Stein GA, Koffman M, et al. Femoral varus-derotation osteotomy in spastic cerebral palsy. J Bone Joint Surg Am 1985;67:1229–35.

[129] Black BE, Griffin PP. The cerebral palsied hip. Clin Orthop Relat Res 1997;42–51.

[130] McCarthy JJ, Betz RR. Hip disorders in children who have spinal cord injury. Orthop Clin North Am 2006;37:197–202.

[131] Han M, Kim H. Chronic hip instability as a cause of autonomic dysreflexia: successful management by resection arthroplasty: a case report. J Bone Joint Surg Am 2003;85:126–8.

[132] Beck M, Woo A, Leunig M, et al. Gluteus minimus-induced femoral head deformation in dysplasia of the hip. Acta Orthop Scand 2001;72:13–7.

[133] Kim HT, Wenger DR. Location of acetabular deficiency and associated hip dislocation in neuromuscular hip dysplasia: three-dimensional computed tomographic analysis. J Pediatr Orthop 1997;17:143–51.

[134] Hubbard AM, Dormans JP. Evaluation of developmental dysplasia, Perthes disease, and neuromuscular dysplasia of the hip in children before and after surgery: an imaging update. AJR Am J Roentgenol 1995;164:1067–73.

[135] Weinstein SL, Mubarak SJ, Wenger DR. Developmental hip dysplasia and dislocation: part II. Instr Course Lect 2004;53:531–42.

[136] Hankinson J, Morton RE. Use of a lying hip abduction system in children with bilateral cerebral palsy: a pilot study. Dev Med Child Neurol 2002;44:177–80.

[137] Pountney T, Mandy A, Green E, et al. Management of hip dislocation with postural management. Child Care Health Dev 2002;28:179–85.

[138] Krach LE, Kriel RL, Gilmartin RC, et al. Hip status in cerebral palsy after one year of continuous intrathecal baclofen infusion. Pediatr Neurol 2004;30:163–8.

[139] Pidcock FS, Fish DE, Johnson-Greene D, et al. Hip migration percentage in children with cerebral palsy treated with botulinum toxin type A. Arch Phys Med Rehabil 2005;86:431–5.

[140] Boyd RN, Dobson F, Parrott J, et al. The effect of botulinum toxin type A and a variable hip abduction orthosis on gross motor function: a randomized controlled trial. Eur J Neurol 2001;8(Suppl 5):109–19.

[141] Hicdonmez T, Steinbok P, Beauchamp R, et al. Hip joint subluxation after selective dorsal rhizotomy for spastic cerebral palsy. J Neurosurg 2005;103:10–6.

[142] Miller F, Bagg MR. Age and migration percentage as risk factors for progression in spastic hip disease. Dev Med Child Neurol 1995;37:449–55.

[143] Song HR, Carroll NC. Femoral varus derotation osteotomy with or without acetabulo-plasty for unstable hips in cerebral palsy. J Pediatr Orthop 1998;18:62–8.

[144] Stott NS, Piedrahita L. AACPDM: effects of surgical adductor releases for hip subluxation in cerebral palsy: an AACPDM evidence report. Dev Med Child Neurol 2004;46:628–45.

[145] Donaldson WF. Complications in pediatric orthopaedic surgery. N Engl J Med 1995;333: 533–4, 10.1056/NEJM199508243330827.

[146] Roposch A, Wedge JH. An incomplete periacetabular osteotomy for treatment of neuro-muscular hip dysplasia. Clin Orthop Relat Res 2005;166–75.

[147] McNerney NP, Mubarak SJ, Wenger DR. One-stage correction of the dysplastic hip in ce-rebral palsy with the San Diego acetabuloplasty: results and complications in 104 hips. J Pediatr Orthop 2000;20:93–103.

[148] Bagg MR, Farber J, Miller F. Long-term follow-up of hip subluxation in cerebral palsy patients. J Pediatr Orthop 1993;13:32–6.

[149] Handelsman JE, Weinberg J, Razi A, et al. The role of AO external fixation in proximal femoral osteotomies in the pediatric neuromuscular population [see comment]. J Pediatr Orthop B 2004;13:303–7.

[150] Thompson CE, Larsen LJ. Recurrent hip dislocation in intermediate spinal atrophy. J Pediatr Orthop 1990;10:638–41.

ELSEVIER
SAUNDERS

Phys Med Rehabil Clin N Am
19 (2008) 195–203

PHYSICAL MEDICINE
AND REHABILITATION
CLINICS OF
NORTH AMERICA

Index

Note: Page numbers of article titles are in **boldface** type.

Moving?

Make sure your subscription moves with you!

To notify us of your new address, find your **Clinics Account Number** (located on your mailing label above your name), and contact customer service at:

E-mail: elspcs@elsevier.com

800-654-2452 (subscribers in the U.S. & Canada)
407-345-4000 (subscribers outside of the U.S. & Canada)

Fax number: 407-363-9661

Elsevier Periodicals Customer Service
6277 Sea Harbor Drive
Orlando, FL 32887-4800

*To ensure uninterrupted delivery of your subscription, please notify us at least 4 weeks in advance of move.